read for patients, providers, and all those taking care of individuals with IBD. "

—**William H. Holderman, MD**, Medical Director,
Digestive Health Specialists, Tacoma, WA

"Lois Fink's book, *Courage Take Guts: Lessons Learned from a Lost Colon*, a truly inspirational story, grabbed my attention from the first chapter. She was able to take me on her extraordinary journey with Crohn's disease, sharing very personal feelings. For people who have or will have ostomy surgery, this is the book to read. Having had ostomy surgery myself, with the diagnosis of ulcerative colitis, this inspirational book would have assisted me in my recovery. Lois reveals how she has made her life worth living, even in the darkest of times. Lois gives patients and their families information on support systems that will assist in their journey to recovery. Thank you, Lois, for sharing your courageous story, and for your selfless dedication to the ostomy community."

—**Susan Burns**, President, United Ostomy Associations
of America (UOAA)

COURAGE TAKES GUTS

Lessons Learned from a Lost Colon

LOIS FINK

First Edition
ISBN-13: 978-1544290874
ISBN-10: 154429087X

Library of Congress Catalog Number: 2016920882

For my late dad, Paul Melvin Fink, survivor of the invasion of Normandy on Omaha Beach during World War II.

His words, said to me so long ago when I was a frightened and terrified teen who had just been diagnosed with Crohn's disease, not only proved true, but continue to inspire me:

"Perhaps one day you will meet someone, and because of what you're going through now, you will know what to say and how to help."

In memory of Cheryl F. "Roni" Baker and Nancy Corene Hekkleman.

Contents

Foreword   i

Acknowledgments   iv

CHAPTER 1

Waiting to Become a Woman   1

CHAPTER 2

Doctors and Padded Bras   4

CHAPTER 3

Why Me?   10

CHAPTER 4

No Boobs to Hold the Dress Up   17

CHAPTER 5

The Mile-High City . . . and Other Lows   20

CHAPTER 6

It's Not Gas, It's a Bowel Obstruction!   26

CHAPTER 7

My Secret: Bowel Incontinence   28

CHAPTER 8

Who Knew Seattle Had Hills?   31

CHAPTER 9

Confronting Ostomy Surgery   35

CHAPTER 10

Stoma 101   39

CHAPTER 11

The Night before Ostomy Surgery   44

CHAPTER 12

Freedom from Fear   51

CHAPTER 13

New Adventures in Seattle   54

CHAPTER 14

Lois Goes to Washington . . . Olympia, Washington   64

CHAPTER 15

What about Intimacy?   70

CHAPTER 16

In the End: Insights Gained   74

ADDITIONAL PERSPECTIVES

What I Know for Sure: Thoughts from an Ostomy Nurse and Patient   80

Serving a Unique Community   88

FURTHER LEARNING

Glossary   97

List of Resources   102

About the Author   111

Speaking Engagements   112

Foreword

Lois was my patient, and then she became my teacher.

I met Lois in the mid-1990s, a few years after finishing my family-medicine residency and starting a practice in Seattle. Lois was a vibrant, energetic woman with many interests. She was well traveled. She had an interesting job. She was a fabulous storyteller with a marvelous sense of humor. And she had Crohn's disease, a serious inflammatory disorder that can affect the entire gastrointestinal tract. By the time I met Lois she was thirty-six, and Crohn's disease was not something that presented a problem in her daily life because she'd had ostomy surgery, a procedure to remove the diseased bowel and create an opening for waste at the abdominal wall.

As with most patients who have chronic conditions, Lois knew a lot about her illness. Young doctors learn from their "patient experts," and I learned from Lois. One of the first things I learned was that she was someone who must be heard. Her path from critically-ill Crohn's patient to healthy woman was often obstructed by doctors who wouldn't listen to her, and if they did listen, they didn't hear or believe what she told them. Her symptoms were attributed to nerves, anxiety, or a psychological problem. Lois's experiences taught me some of my most important lessons about both Crohn's disease and patient care.

In 2002, after being her doctor for a number of years, I asked Lois if she had ever considered speaking to medical or nursing students. She had just written a chapter for Rolf Benirschke's book, *Great Comebacks from Ostomy Surgery,* and I was so impressed with her passion and expertise that I suggested she contact the medical school. I warned her that the curriculum was packed and it might not be easy to convince the school to add her to the lecture schedule, but encouraged her to find a way to share her experience with medical students. "That's your assignment," I told her.

Lois loved the idea that it might be possible to educate young doctors and nurses about Crohn's disease from the patient perspective: about how ostomy surgery could be a positive and life-changing intervention, and mostly, how important it is for health-care professionals to listen to their patients.

Lois took my suggestion to call the local medical school, and I soon learned that she doesn't do anything on the small scale. Soon, she was lecturing to medical students and then to nursing students. She began working with ostomy supply companies, and then with ostomy nurses, as a speaker and advocate, and she also started presenting at professional conferences. She wrote articles about Crohn's disease and ostomy surgery for local and national publications and appeared on radio talk shows. She worked on projects with Mike McCready, the lead guitarist for Pearl Jam who also has Crohn's and is an advocate and activist. In short, she rocks.

Advocacy and education weren't enough for Lois. She contacted her state representative about creating a bathroom-access bill for people with Crohn's disease. She worked with her representative, testified before the state legislature, and got a law passed in 2009. In 2011, along with a colleague, she created an IBD and Ostomy Awareness ribbon. Using her matchless skill for wordsmithing and bathroom humor, Lois came up with the tagline, "It's more than a ribbon, it's a movement."

Before Lois received a correct diagnosis and treatment, her symptoms were downplayed, trivialized, or simply misunderstood. She felt she didn't have a voice. Hers is the story of a woman who not only persisted in getting the care she needed, but who believed her story could help others. Lois found her voice and fearlessly raised it, teaching health professionals, legislators, community leaders, and her doctor.

—Deborah E. Klein, MD, Swedish Physicians,
Seattle, WA

Acknowledgments

This book would not have been possible without the generous support of Susan Balmas, Denise Barbour, Chris Bergerson, Barbara Berk, Joanne Cohen, Sarah Christensen, Linda Feldman, Zane Fink, Tina Kirk, Sue Ellen Klein, Ellen Pierce, Richard Schiller, Alan I. Segal, David Segall, Jacob Segall, Douglas Stocks, Gail Taback, and Pamela Tauman. Thank you to Markley Motors, Inc. as well.

To my friends in Seattle, Fort Collins, and Littleton who encouraged and supported me in countless ways. You know who you are!

To Lois Hart, my "book mentor," who shared her knowledge, expertise, and time, and who believed in me when I doubted I could ever write this book.

To Molly McCowan of Inkbot Editing, who came into my life when I needed her and fine-tuned my book with her skillful editing and professional formatting.

To Rebecca Finkel of F+P Graphic Design, who took the existing front and back cover designs and made them snap.

To Judith Briles, the "Book Shepherd," whose class on publishing at a Northern Colorado Writers conference convinced me that I should and could self-publish. Her help and support were invaluable.

To Joanna Burgess, Certified Wound, Ostomy, and Continence Nurse (CWOCN®), whose suggestions and insights were always on point. Joanna's friendship, both personal and professional, has enriched my life in countless ways.

To Computer Resource in Fort Collins, especially Michael Stolz and Carol Howard, for their time, help, and hand-holding!

ACKNOWLEDGMENTS

To Gail Wodzin, of Gail Ann Photography, for her continued support and talented skills, both on my website and in capturing my spirit in her photos.

To Nancy Leff, who was a true friend in those dark beginning years after my diagnosis of Crohn's disease. Everyone needs a friend who can jokingly say (and with a straight face), "She's into bottoms."

To my English teacher at Taylor Allderdice High School, Mrs. Lewis, who said, "You should be a writer."

To the countless medical and nursing students at the University of Washington, Seattle University, the University of Colorado Anschutz Medical Campus, and the University of Northern Colorado for encouraging me to write my story. I'm glad I finally listened to them!

To everyone struggling with Crohn's disease or facing ostomy surgery, you are not alone and you do not have to be ashamed or embarrassed because you have a bowel disease or a stoma. Ostomy surgery can be the beginning of a new life and an opportunity for personal growth and development. It all depends on how you choose to view your situation. I hope sharing my story gives you strength and courage.

You *can* live life to the fullest without a colon or rectum!

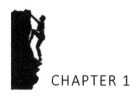

CHAPTER 1

Waiting to Become a Woman

Who doesn't love a good movie complete with gripping plot, strong characters, and a satisfying ending? Of course, a warm bag of buttered, salted popcorn makes the experience even more satisfying.

Aside from *Sleeping Beauty*, *Lady and the Tramp*, and *Cinderella*, the one movie that made a strong impression on my twelve-year-old mind was the film I saw in sixth grade about that magical time of "becoming a woman."

Becoming a Woman was filled with soft-but-stirring musical numbers about the time our bodies will change because of something called "hormones." I always wondered what a hormone looked like. The film never featured a close-up of these mystical entities. After these tiny substances circulated through our bodies, our breasts would develop and we'd experience the first of many menstrual periods. We would magically produce blood that would appear in our panties in what resembled a butterfly! This abstract picture would signal that we were on our way to becoming a woman. I had to blink several times once the lights came on in the classroom because my mind kept thinking about what pattern I'd find in my panties.

Seemingly overnight, my girlfriends had budding breasts and wore training bras designed to stretch. Then, as their breasts grew larger, they graduated to regular bras. I, on the other hand, appeared to be a late bloomer. I could wear a training bra, but there was nothing to train! I thought long and hard about how to speed up this womanhood process. Although my maternal grandmother (my *bubbe*, which is Yiddish for grandmother and pronounced "bub-bee"), with whom I'd had a special bond, had died when I was in fourth grade, I still sensed her presence. Many times at night, I shared my triumphs and struggles with her. Figuring Bubbe Leah would understand, I directed my prayers to the God who had parted the Red Sea for my ancestors as they fled Egypt. This profound miracle, retold yearly at every Passover Seder, had made a strong impression on my mind. If God could accomplish this, surely invoking my menstrual period would be considered a minor feat on the miracle meter.

Even at a young age, I was task-oriented. In addition to praying, I decided that positive action could also play a role in my becoming a woman. I realized that if I walked slightly bent over, the front of my blouse or shirtwaist dress would balloon out, giving the illusion of breast development. I walked hunched over by day and prayed to God for my period to arrive by night. *Hunch over, pray at night, wait and wait.* The hoped-for miracle never happened. I consoled myself by thinking that perhaps God had more pressing matters at hand and would check back with me later.

By fourteen, my weight had topped the scale between eighty and eighty-five pounds. Because I had a poor appetite, my parents began bribing me with free use of what used to be known as a department-store card. You brought the card and a note from your parents to the designated store and purchased what you wanted. (This was the era before Visa and MasterCard. Today, if a parent gave a teenager use of their credit card or Amazon account, they'd be filing for bankruptcy within the hour.)

"If you just get to ninety pounds, you can buy that powder-blue, cable-knit Mohair wool sweater all your girlfriends are wearing," my mom announced. But I couldn't get my weight up to ninety pounds, and besides, I didn't care about clothes. They hung shapelessly on my bony body and I hated looking in the mirror.

"Look at you," my mother would say. "You're nothing but skin and bones. Why won't you eat? What am I going to do with you?"

Thoughts of becoming a woman ceased being important. I didn't have an answer for my mother or myself as to why I didn't want to eat and why I looked the way I did. Instead, I began hating myself, along with the image in the mirror that stared back at me.

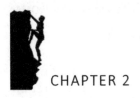

CHAPTER 2

Doctors and Padded Bras

One of the hallmarks of a good doctor is really listening to the patient and then piecing together symptoms to come up with an accurate diagnosis, instead of blaming the patient when the cause of the illness isn't easily identifiable.

Our family doctor made frequent house calls to see me when I was fifteen. In fact, every six weeks he would announce that my abdominal pain, fever, and diarrhea were the result of a stomach virus. He prescribed phenobarbital to dull the pain. He never seemed puzzled by the persistent, unrelenting ailment.

With my weight staying between eighty and eighty-five pounds, along with my arrested breast development, my mother decided to take action in the form of padded bras. I hated wearing them; they reminded me I wasn't "normal." Pointy and hard, the bra cups resembled the ends of a Red Delicious apple! But the fear of not looking like my girlfriends overpowered my anger, and I reluctantly wore them. Frustration went underground at that point, and expressed itself in my refusal to regularly wash the bras. My mother then threatened to take them from me. Reluctantly, I agreed to keep them clean. The anger I felt for these "padded apples" reflected my increasing self-loathing.

Changing for high school gym class caused my anxiety to rise to a new level. While changing, I would use the open door of the locker as a shield to hide my prepubescent chest and the despised bra. Like gym class, swimming lessons were mandatory. Panicked, I pleaded with one family physician to write a note saying I suffered from sinusitis and could not attend swimming. The embarrassment of wearing the all-revealing one-piece suit and the inevitable ridicule I'd be subjected to had me in a state of anxiety until the doctor relented and wrote the note. Teenage girls have a talent for cruelty that teen boys can't even begin to rival.

At sixteen, I still had no signs of menstruation or breast development, and my mother, alarmed I might never have children, called for an exam by her gynecologist. My bearing children was important to my mother. Perhaps it signaled to her circle of friends and the larger Jewish community where I grew up that she had fulfilled her role as a mother by instilling in me the importance of having children. She looked forward to the day when she would be called Bubbe Ann. But giving birth was not on my radar. The idea of a gynecological exam terrified me. I was already aware that my body didn't look "normal."

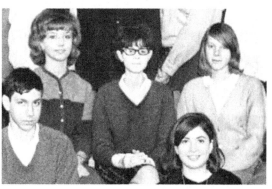

Me at Taylor Allderdice High School (center).

Self-conscious and embarrassed, I even wondered if I was in some way responsible for my lack of physical development. I wanted to ask my mom what would happen when the doctor examined me, but I sensed her reluctance to broach the topic. After the examination, the gynecologist assured us that my birth canal looked normal; I would be able to bear children, but he couldn't explain why my ovaries were not maturing. His diagnosis, while perhaps giving my mother some comfort, only heightened my underlying sense of anxiety that I wasn't "normal."

As the knife-like abdominal pain intensified, the diarrhea occurred with increasing regularity and tormented me day and night. I also experienced leg cramps, which I later found out were due to the lack of potassium and other vital electrolytes caused by my compromised gastrointestinal tract.

My mother, now alarmed and anxious, took me to numerous physicians. After each examination, the diagnosis was the same: *No physical basis for the patient's symptoms.* My leg cramps were written off as growing pains! But I wasn't growing. Instead, I felt trapped in perpetual prepubescence. We consulted a gastroenterologist, and he determined I needed a sigmoidoscopy. Today, the scopes are soft and flexible. That was not the case in the mid-1960s. Today, you lie on your side for the examination, but I knelt on a stool with my derriere pointing up as the doctor roughly maneuvered the scope. Once again, my symptoms were curtly dismissed. He declared nothing physically wrong with me, only that I was a nervous child. "If you don't watch it," he warned, "you'll be a good candidate for colitis."

After this brutal examination, I told my mother I would no longer see any more doctors. They were dismissive, had no compassion, and didn't listen to me.

I didn't tell my mother that the abdominal pain had become so severe that I'd nearly pass out in between classes during school. I'd slump against the wall, fighting the urge to faint from the pain's vice-like grip. Sweat would dot my forehead while stars danced in front of my eyes.

In the early 1960s, when a doctor told a parent that there was nothing physically wrong with their child, there was no further discussion. My mother decided it was time to have a serious discussion with me about my health. She explained that numerous specialists all had come to the same conclusion that there was nothing physically wrong with me.

"You have to get a grip on yourself, Lois," she said. "If you don't, I'm afraid you're going to end up in a hospital, and it's not going to be a normal one. Do you understand what I'm trying to tell you?"

I assured my mother that I understood. I was running the risk of being admitted to a mental hospital. I sat at my little vanity in my bedroom, and when my mom left, I stared into the oval mirror. "There is nothing physically wrong with you, Lois," I said. "All the doctors have said the same thing." I repeated those words over and over, watching myself in the mirror. Then, something rebelled inside. "I'm not making this up. There *is* something wrong." At a gut level, I knew I was very sick.

My illness only accentuated the normal friction between mother and daughter during the volatile teenage years. At the time, I didn't realize how frustrated and powerless my mother felt. The medical experts had decreed that my symptoms were all in my head. My mother was trapped in the medical nightmare just as much as I was; the quandary between wanting to believe me and deferring to the medical experts must have been unbearable.

Shortly after my seventeenth birthday, my symptoms intensified and I started losing weight at an alarming rate. I was constantly thirsty. The sight and smell of food nauseated me. Because the diarrhea tormented me day and night, I grew more and more malnourished, was in constant pain, and suffered from sleep deprivation.

A mass had developed in the lower-right quadrant of my abdomen, and with every step I took, I felt it quivering. I made a detached, self-diagnosis of cancer. My thinking was very linear and straightforward: *a mass equals cancer equals death*. I calculated that I would die within the next few months. There was no point in telling anyone because no one would listen, and I couldn't handle another doctor telling me I was conjuring up my symptoms.

At my mother's pleading, I agreed to be seen by one final physician. While in the examination room, I developed a fever of 102 degrees. "Lois, you can't manufacture fevers at will," the doctor said. "There is something wrong with you, and we have to run tests to figure out what it is."

I shouted, "No, you aren't coming near me!" This was the only doctor who had ever really listened and looked at me, but I'd had it with tests. He suspected either Crohn's disease or ulcerative colitis, and he arranged a time with my parents to run a barium series during my spring break.

But the Crohn's disease hidden in the shadow of my small bowel wasn't content to wait for me to undergo medical testing. In February of my senior year, as I began the long trek up the steep hill toward home after school, I shifted my weight to the left side of my body so I wouldn't feel the roiling mass as much. By the time I walked in the door, I knew I'd reached the end of my endurance. I collapsed on the couch and said, "Mom, I can't go on anymore."

With a vengeance, pain assaulted my body, doubling me over. Sweat beaded up on my forehead. My mother took one look at my contorted face and called yet another doctor. When he pressed his hands down on the lower-right section of my abdomen and then quickly lifted them up, I screamed in agony. Turning slowly toward my anxious mother, he pronounced matter-of-factly, "She has appendicitis."

My mother's parents were born in Eastern Europe; her mother in Russia and her father in Romania. Due to poverty and poor nutrition, they were small in stature, like many of their peers. My mom topped the height chart at four foot ten. But what she lacked in stature, she more than made up for in righteous indignation.

Black eyes blazing with laser precision directed at the unsuspecting physician, she hurled, "You mean to tell me my daughter has had appendicitis for nearly two years and the medical profession is just figuring this out?"

His silence was deafening. He finally muttered, "Do you know any surgeons?"

Even through the haze of pain, I clearly saw my mother's anger. Sheer willpower on my mother's part saved the hapless physician from bodily harm.

I was rushed to the local hospital and prepped for an emergency appendectomy, which, instead of a swollen appendix, revealed a badly inflamed portion of the ileum, the last section of the small bowel. Because of the severe inflammation, proceeding further would have risked a massive infection.

I was about to learn what had been tormenting my body for nearly two years.

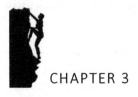

CHAPTER 3

Why Me?

Being diagnosed with a chronic, incurable disease isn't easy. Our first thoughts are shock, denial, and *Why me?* The answer to that question would serve as a road map for me later in my life, but it would be years before I would learn that my diagnosis was a gift.

As I concentrated on the indignation of being on the children's floor of Montefiore Hospital in Pittsburgh, having to abide by rules I didn't feel pertained to me, a doctor walked into the room, interrupting my thoughts of circumventing the regulations posted on the hospital-room door.

Dr. Chamovitz introduced himself as a gastroenterologist. Instantly, I was on guard as memories of the brutal treatment I'd received at the hands of the previous specialist came flooding back.

"You don't have appendicitis. You have Crohn's disease," he said flatly. I remember those four paralyzing words from fifty years ago as if it were yesterday.

I briefly felt a smug sense of satisfaction that quickly gave way to fear. In 1966, Crohn's disease wasn't on the public's health radar. I didn't like the sound of that diagnosis. It seemed more suitable for an old person, and I was a sophisticated seventeen-year-old, even if I looked like a prepubescent girl. I wasn't about to let details get in my way. I pushed away panic that threatened to overtake me by concentrating on the words coming out of the doctor's mouth: "Do you notice anything different?"

It took a while before I could answer. "This is the first night I've spent without pain in a long while."

"Do you want to know why?" he asked. Of course I wanted to know why. Was he dim-witted?

He pointed to the needle in my arm and explained that I was receiving intravenous steroid medication to quiet the inflammation. The doctors needed to know how much of my small bowel was diseased, and whether or not there was colonic involvement. The standard tests back then were a barium small-bowel follow-through and a barium enema. These tests outlined the small and large intestines with a thin film of barium that showed up on radiographs and helped to define the areas of bowel that were normal in diameter versus narrowed and diseased.

Swallowing the chalky barium, no matter how much Hershey's chocolate syrup was added to mask the thick, viscous liquid, resulted in bouts of choking. The test took hours as the barium slowly made its way through the upper gastrointestinal tract and x-rays were taken at key intervals.

As unpleasant as drinking the barium was, it didn't compare to the humiliation of the barium enemas. The technician was usually male, and even with a female attendant present, I was mortified as an enema was inserted into my anus, causing barium to flow into my rectum and slowly throughout my colon. Again, x-rays were taken at specified points along the colonic route. The technician would say, "Hold still . . . don't breathe . . . okay, you can breathe."

My body would be maneuvered into different positions for the x-rays, and I was keenly aware of the rubber tubing extending out of my rectum and between my legs. I made every effort to keep my hospital gown closed in the back as much as possible, but I was still mortified. Hot tears would stream down my face as I waited for the awful test to be over.

I spent three weeks in the hospital struggling to come to terms with my diagnosis. Doctors deemed my physical, emotional, and psychological health as too precarious and I was not allowed to return to school, which added to my feelings of isolation. I was homeschooled for the remaining four months of my senior year.

Shortly after the diagnosis, my mom found a small article about Suzanne Rosenthal, a New Yorker who also had Crohn's disease. Her husband and friends were laying the groundwork for a foundation that would raise funds to find a cause and cure for Crohn's disease and ulcerative colitis. I carried that article with me for a year. It became my only link to someone who had gone through what I was experiencing. It helped me feel not quite so alone.

"Why me?" I angrily hurled the words at my father. I doubted my dad would have a credible answer. Most teenagers come to the conclusion that their parents know very little, and I was no exception. My father was one of the few individuals who survived the initial invasion of Normandy on Omaha Beach during World War II. He relayed everything in military terms, and to my way of thinking, he was clueless. I didn't realize that he felt equally as powerless as my mom did, and that he also struggled with discussing this bowel disease with me. "I don't know," he began.

Why did I even bother asking, I thought ruefully.

"Perhaps later in life," he continued, "you will meet someone, and because of what you're going through now, you will know what to say and how to help." I stared in disbelief upon hearing those words.

It would be years before I fully understood the power of my father's answer. They continue to inspire me, and I maintain a connection with him even though his life ended in 1994.

Treatment with prednisone caused my body to swell with fluid, resulting in the classic "moon face." Overnight, I'd morphed into a chipmunk! Staring in a mirror at my swollen face, I thought the only things missing were the fur and tail. Steroids can cause a temporary increase in facial hair, so my description wasn't too far off. I felt like a caricature of myself, and confided to a cousin that I was embarrassed for friends to see me. Swollen ankles made walking difficult. Weekly diuretic shots to help my body eliminate the excess fluid were ineffective. Emotional swings accentuated my feelings of frustration, and at times I doubted my hold on reality.

Adding to the angst of dealing with the side effects of the drug was the special diet I had to follow. It was easier for me to detail what I *could* eat because the list of what I couldn't eat was too lengthy. My appetite was returning and I wanted to eat everything I was allowed, not because the disease was being controlled, but because the steroids stimulated my appetite. I became an efficient eating machine, but could never feel satiated. I gained weight, but it was all in the form of fluid. Not only was my face round like the moon, but my entire body felt bloated. What I craved was a normal "teenager's diet" consisting of pizza, hot dogs, french fries, soda, spicy food, fried chicken, fresh fruits, and anything with seeds— everything I was not allowed to have.

Being a resourceful teen, I was not about to let this diet completely rob me of time with my friends, so I figured out a way to go out for a "burger." It's true, seeds were one of the food groups not allowed to grace my mouth. After careful examination of the hamburger's mate, the bun, I came up with a plan I was confident would work. Now it was time for a trial run. My friend Nancy joined me at the local hamburger hut. When it was time to place my order, I requested two *bottom* buns. The puzzled employee looked at me askance and asked me to repeat myself.

"I'd like my hamburger on two bottom buns," I said nonchalantly, as if this request were commonplace. For several seconds, we stared at each other.

"Give my friend the bottom bun on my order and I'll take her top half." The perplexed server shook her head, trying to process my request, and finally complied. I flashed her a wide grin. Leaning over the counter, Nancy casually said, "She's secretly into bottoms. Don't argue with her!"

The top half of the bun is littered with sesame seeds, but the bottom half of the bun has far fewer, and they were much easier to pick out. When my order came, I carefully turned the bottom half of the bun over, picked out the targeted seeds one by one, and proceeded to enjoy my burger. Dreaded diet be damned!

Though I'd scored a victory against sesame seeds, I couldn't join my classmates at Mineo's Pizza House on Fridays after school. As much as I loved pizza, I couldn't figure out how to remove the spicy tomato sauce, and I was forced to concede defeat when it came to Italian food.

Three months after my diagnosis, I found myself back in the hospital experiencing a major flare-up, despite the steroid therapy. This time, multiple doctors tried to determine why my secondary growth and development had been arrested. I was poked, peered at, and discussed as if I wasn't present. I felt invisible and demeaned, like I was a new life form being studied under a microscope. I wanted to shout "I'm here! I can hear you! Stop talking about me!" as they stared at my prepubescent body and scribbled notes.

I had regular visits with Dr. Chamovitz; he looked a little like Robert Redford, but I wasn't about to let him know I thought he was cute! I still felt very scared and angry, and I resented having to wear a bathing suit in order to get my picture taken for my chart. It took several years before I warmed up to him. The one valuable lesson I learned from Dr. Chamovitz was that I had a right to a physician who would talk to me, answer my questions, and explain why he was performing certain tests. "If you have a doctor who won't do this, you have every right to find another one," he said.

After five months on high doses of prednisone, there was no sign of the disease going into remission. When surgery was recommended, my parents wanted a second opinion. There were few experts on Crohn's disease in Pittsburgh at that time, so my mother and I flew to Philadelphia to see Dr. Chamovitz's mentor. This meant having to go through the upper and lower GI tests yet again. Time did not soften the embarrassment and degradation of the experience.

After reviewing the current test results and comparing them with the previous ones, he also recommended surgery, specifically a bowel resection. It would be the only way for me to have a normal life. He looked at me and said, "Go home, have the surgery, and *zai a mensch.*" He asked if I knew what he had said.

"Of course I know what you said," I replied. "I know some Yiddish! I'm Jewish!" Roughly translated, a *mensch* is the personification of worth and dignity requiring the highest respect; an upright, honorable person. He wanted me to "be a healthy human being."

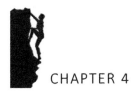

CHAPTER 4

No Boobs to Hold the Dress Up

The prom is an important rite of passage that brings back wonderful memories for so many people, no matter how many years have passed. When facing a chronic illness and major surgery, however, a high school event takes the back seat. Fear was the partner I danced with.

The night before I was to have my first bowel resection was also the evening of my senior prom. My mom and I sat on the front porch and watched my friend Robbie step out in a beautiful formal gown, escorted by her father. My mother never finished high school. She had to stop in the tenth grade to go to work and help support the family. My *zeyde* (Yiddish for grandfather) did little to earn a living, being content to sit and read scholarly books for a good part of the day. He would have made an excellent rabbi.

While my mother lamented the fact that I couldn't experience this important rite of passage, I spent the time thinking about my upcoming surgery. Despite this, I still had to resist the urge to yell, "Ma, I don't even have the boobs to hold the dress up! I don't care about the prom." Crohn's disease had eclipsed everything.

The bowel resection resulted in six inches of my small intestine and a foot and a half of my large intestine (colon) being removed. Surgeons removed the diseased section of the bowel and sutured the two ends together. The surgery was a success, and I recovered quickly. For the first time in years, I could enjoy a normal life. I gained weight rapidly and my secondary growth blossomed. The anticipated wait to "become a woman" had finally materialized! I learned that when Crohn's disease is active during puberty, secondary growth and development can be delayed. Suddenly, the puzzle of my wayward development was solved.

I began my freshman year at Duquesne University, and it felt good to be alive. For the first time, I became acutely aware of how wonderful it felt to breathe, to see the vibrant colors of summer, to hear the birds singing, to watch and listen to the rustling of leaves in the wind. Being able to have food again was a delight. I remember the day I ate a fuzzy, juicy peach, its sun-ripened juice dripping from my mouth.

My recovery was short-lived. Nearly one year to the day after my first bowel resection, the fevers, diarrhea, and weight loss returned. "We don't know a lot about Crohn's disease," Dr. Chamovitz told me, "but we do know it keeps recurring." Admitted to the hospital again, I had to curtail most of my college classes. At least this time I wasn't on the children's floor.

I began a regimen that would continue for the next five years: high doses of steroids, minimum attendance at college, and the restrictive diet. Subduing the disease seemed to take forever. Depression linked hands with Crohn's disease and encircled me in a deep chasm. I would sit for hours, unable to see past the thick, dark wall that separated me from the rest of the world.

Sensing my need for comfort, Colonel, my German shepherd, would sit next to me, his head resting in my lap while salty tears rolled down my face, wetting us both. Echoes of laughter broke through the depressed stupor when I watched Red Skelton and Jonathan Winters on television. Somehow, I held on. With what felt like glacial speed, the inflammation in my GI tract gradually quieted, and the fevers and pain dissipated.

It took five years to complete college, but I graduated with a degree in elementary education. My proud parents looked on as I received my degree. Even the black armband I wore protesting the Vietnam conflict didn't dampen my dad's elation at seeing his daughter achieve a goal that at one time seemed unobtainable.

It was time to finally begin living my life. Two weeks after graduation, I hugged my parents and Colonel and then boarded a plane for the city I'd dreamed about living in since I was eight years old: Denver, Colorado. The Mile-High City.

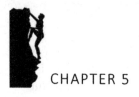

CHAPTER 5

The Mile-High City . . . and Other Lows

When you graduate from college you feel invincible, like Superwoman. At least that's how I felt, along with having a healthy dose of anything-is-possible. We need to bottle this feeling and have it available to inhale when life's tough times threaten to undermine our belief in ourselves.

I landed in Denver's Stapleton International Airport in early June 1971, and proceeded to locate the nearest YWCA. I figured a young Jewish lady would be safe there. After checking in and hanging up my clothes, I decided to explore the area around the "hotel." Everything seemed larger than life and much brighter than dark, cramped Pittsburgh. The view of the snowcapped, jagged Rocky Mountains nearly took my breath away. I watched bemusedly as people walked diagonally across the downtown intersections. That did not happen in Pittsburgh! Maybe it had something to do with the mile-high altitude.

The next morning, I found the municipal building that housed the Teacher Placement Service Department, which advertised that if you agreed to teach west of Denver, they would do the legwork necessary to find a position for you. I envisioned myself in Aspen, Breckenridge, or any of the other fascinating places on the Western Slope.

When I was in my last semester of college, I'd

come out to Denver and interviewed with various school districts. Based on the information I'd learned then, I came to the conclusion that my best opportunity of gaining employment was with the Jefferson County School District.

I planned my strategy. This consisted of finding out the name of the superintendent's assistant and getting to know her over the phone. After introducing myself, I asked her how her weekend had been and let her know how much I wanted to work in the Jefferson County district. I did this every Monday morning. How could she resist my endearing charm?

While I waited for my plan to bear fruit, I took a position at a local daycare center. While it didn't lend itself to actual teaching, I was determined to be gainfully employed while I awaited the position I really wanted. A girl has to make a living!

I also knew I wanted a more permanent living situation than the YWCA. I was put in touch with two women looking for a roommate, and I set up a time to meet. The timing was perfect. The day before our meeting, I watched in horror as a cockroach scuttled across the floor of my room at the YWCA. My entire body shuddered. "I wasn't raised to live with roaches," I yelled at the top of my lungs. "I'm getting out tomorrow." That's exactly what I did.

When you move in with two women who've known each other since childhood, guess who ends up being the odd woman out? Anxious to make a good impression on my new housemates, I cooked dinner for all of us that first night. Sitting at the dining-room table and making polite chitchat, I noticed Rose looking intently at me. "What nationality are you?" she barked. I instantly knew where this line of questioning was headed.

"American," I said.

I could see this wasn't the answer Rose wanted. She asked it again. I repeated my answer slowly, enunciating my words. By now, my new roommate was clearly testy, and I decided to proceed with discretion. Rose wanted to know my religion. Any Jewish person who's asked the "nationality" question knows they are likely dealing with someone who is not open-minded about religion. I finally told her I was Jewish and found out she'd been raised in a strict Catholic home. "That's great," I muttered.

Six weeks later, I discovered how Rose felt about cohabitation with a Jewish woman. I was informed I could no longer ride in her car, watch her television, or use her ironing board. She'd designated small sections in the kitchen cabinets and refrigerator for my food; the rest of the storage space was for her and Glenny. It had been years since I'd encountered anti-Semitism, and it hurt, deeply. I moved out within the week.

I heard about a woman looking to share her modern two-bedroom, two-bath apartment. Upon moving in, I soon realized she had an unnatural relationship with her pet parakeet. I had to resist the urge to shudder visibly when the bird would take a few steps into her mouth as she talked. Was there such a dish as parakeet tartare? Her strict rules of no dishes left in the sink, keeping my bedroom neat and orderly, and never allowing my belongings to grace her walls or living room were too constricting.

I finally found a place of my own. Even though I only had used furniture and a bookcase made from cinder blocks, it didn't matter. I was blissfully alone! In addition to having a succession of roommates, I also had a series of jobs, from working in the daycare center to selling shoes in an upscale Denver department store, to finally being able to teach. My persistence in contacting the superintendent's assistant paid off, and after selling shoes for six weeks, a skill I never mastered, I received a call to be a part-time teacher for third-grade students. I was ecstatic. It didn't matter that I would only earn $210 a month (my apartment cost $105 a month). I could finally work in the profession I'd gone to school for, live where I'd dreamed of since I was a child, and listen to John Denver sing "Rocky Mountain High" on the radio.

Being a part-time teacher, I didn't have a contract. So, by the end of the school year, I found myself once again unemployed. In June of 1972, I received a call from the Teacher Placement Service notifying me of a position west of Denver. I was overjoyed. Visions of Aspen and Breckenridge danced in my head, complete with sparkling snow. Then the voice said Uravan. "Ura-what?" I replied.

Uravan, it turned out, was the Union Carbide Corporation's company town, located 103 miles southwest of Grand Junction, pretty much in the middle of nowhere. This little town had fewer than 1,000 residents, and mined uranium and vanadium. Put the two together and you get Uravan. The superintendent of the area wanted to know if I'd ever lived in a small town before. "Of course," I told him. "Denver. It's smaller than Pittsburgh." I had no idea what I was getting myself into when I agreed to the interview.

On hearing that I was heading out for an interview with the superintendent, my dad decided that his little girl shouldn't make the trip by herself, so he flew out and we made the drive together. We arrived in the small town of Naturita around dinnertime and located the only restaurant. Every head turned as we walked in the door. We weren't "town folk," and our clothing announced it even more, especially mine. Even though I'd graduated from college, my way of dressing (wire-rimmed octagonal glasses and navy-blue pea coat) still screamed college student.

During my interview, I learned that because I didn't work for Union Carbide, I couldn't live in Uravan. I had to live in Nucla, another town about the same size as Uravan that was about fifteen miles away.

Finding suitable housing proved challenging. My dad filled the holes in the ceiling of the "spacious house" I'd found with newspaper to stop the heat from escaping. Getting heat from a propane tank located outside was another new experience for me. Luckily, the water didn't come from a well! I rented the house because the kitchen, and all-important bathroom, had been updated.

Word travels fast in rural, small-town America, and my pertinent statistics were communicated to key members of the community, one being the pharmacist. Upon presenting him with my prescription for birth control pills, he said I didn't need them because I was single. I resisted the temptation to counter with a sarcastic retort because I didn't want to alienate anyone or be branded "difficult."

The school building was a metal Quonset hut that had a leaky roof. My classroom was the only room that didn't need coffee cans to catch raindrops, though, so that was a highlight. I also had the opportunity to learn about Navajo culture from one of my Native American students. His grandmother presented me with a beautiful handmade rug that I treasured. Because I had such a small class of seven children, I had the opportunity to teach topics I likely wouldn't have been able to in a structured city classroom. I loved watching my students' faces as they learned new ideas. Despite this, I'd had enough of small-town living, and I counted the days until the school year ended and I could move back to Denver. In the mid-1970s, teaching positions were difficult to find. The mantra for young women of my generation was, "Go into teaching and your future will be mapped out for you." That had become a dead end. After a few interviews, one being in Leadville, another mining town known as "Cloud City" because of its 10,000-foot altitude, I realized it was time to change professions.

I applied for a position with the University of Colorado Medical Center, took a job as a clerk in medical records, and worked my way up through several different positions, one being the receptionist in the child psychiatry clinic. Dealing with the unorganized psychiatrists (and the children and their parents!) and answering a multi-line phone kept me busy.

After working in the clinic for a year, I realized I'd taken the job home. When I answered my home phone with, "Hello, child psychiatry clinic," one day, I knew I probably needed a change of pace.

The popular saying "be careful what you wish for—you might get it," was about to ring true.

CHAPTER 6

It's Not Gas, It's a Bowel Obstruction!

When someone has a history of a bowel disease, people often attribute it to stress. "It's just a little cramping," they say. "All you need to do is relax." How can you relax when it feels like there's a wrench twisting your guts into a knot?

During these years, Crohn's disease was silently planning another major flare-up. My life had been fairly normal for about nine years since my first bowel resection in 1966. I had three to four normal bowel movements a day. I was under the care of a gastroenterologist whom I saw on a regular basis.

In the summer of 1975, the situation changed rapidly. I had been experiencing abdominal pain for about a week, and it had steadily gotten worse. I was used to dealing with occasional diarrhea, but one day I was unable to have any bowel movements, so I grew concerned. My friends kept telling me my abdominal pain stemmed from stress because of the pressures at my job. At a gut level (no pun intended), I knew better. Pain and the cessation of bowel movements for nearly a week had me worried. Could I have a bowel obstruction?

My roommate and I went out to dinner to celebrate the end of the workweek. Halfway through the meal, I felt nauseated. A few hours later, my abdomen became distended and hard. Our neighbor, a physician, diagnosed me over the phone as having a bad attack of gas. As the pain grew worse, I knew my situation was more severe than trapped gas in my intestine, and I asked my roommate to get me to the Rose Medical Center. She drove as fast as she could while I tried to suppress my cries of pain.

A young emergency room resident approached to examine me and I told him if he touched my abdomen, I'd kill him. Pain has a way of making people say irrational things! Doctors admitted me for observation. Initially, they diagnosed me as having an abdominal abscess. I was told that if I didn't undergo another bowel resection, my colon would likely perforate.

Crohn's disease seemed to be gloating. It had been burrowing through my colon like a predator planning an attack on its unsuspecting prey. I knew the drill all too well: high doses of steroids and a restrictive, low-residue diet.

Recovery from the surgery required a six-week hiatus from work. I slept long hours at night and took frequent naps during the day. Recovery seemed to take longer than the first bowel resection. I'd later learn why.

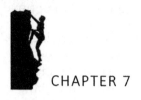

CHAPTER 7

My Secret: Bowel Incontinence

Bowel incontinence. We don't talk about it or want to hear about it. There are television commercials discussing bladder incontinence and "dependable" underwear, usually for women. Diarrhea is nervously laughed about. But bowel incontinence is a divide that remains uncrossed.

Crohn's disease had been insidiously tunneling through my colon and rectum ever since my first flare-up in 1967, relentlessly scarring and narrowing rectal sphincter muscles. This meant that I needed to know the exact location of a bathroom wherever I went. The anxiety over finding a bathroom was nearly unbearable.

I couldn't sit through a movie or enjoy a meal at a restaurant without running to the bathroom several times. I missed a lot of movie plots and ate a lot of cold food! A leisurely walk in the park became a source of extreme anxiety. If I went shopping for clothes, I'd check to see if the fitting rooms were close to the bathroom. There were days when I was "bathroom-bound," stuck at home due to severe diarrhea.

As the disease progressed, I made changes in the kind of clothing I wore. I stopped wearing white, opting for dark-colored clothing. I wouldn't wear shorts. If I had an accident while wearing shorts, everyone around me would know what had happened. In an effort to find humor in what I was going through, I'd joke about my worst nightmare: having to arm wrestle an eighty-year-old woman for a vacant bathroom stall! I reasoned that the elderly usually had issues with constipation, so diarrhea took precedent over slow-moving stool.

When my entire colon and rectum became diseased, I lost control completely and began to experience total bowel incontinence.

Venturing out became emotionally terrifying. I couldn't leave the house without carrying spare underwear and pantyhose. What would I do if the bathroom was occupied? How would I cope with not getting to the bathroom in time and having an accident? How would I conceal it from people around me? I became adept at making jokes. "That'll teach me to look before I sit." Inwardly, I burned crimson from embarrassment.

One day, while shopping at a fashionable department store, I knew I couldn't get to the bathroom in time, and lost control. Keenly aware of the strong odor, I casually walked out of the store as if nothing had happened. I fought for emotional control until my car offered me the escape I needed. Tears nearly blinded me as I drove home, sitting in a pool of hot liquid feces, fighting hard not to vomit from the stench. It seemed to take forever to get home and even longer to feel clean as I sat crying in a bathtub of hot water. Afterward, I wrapped up the soiled jeans in a garbage bag and threw them in the trash. I couldn't wear them again. They were a painful reminder of how Crohn's disease ravaged my body.

Only a few very close friends knew what I was going through. I felt too humiliated and afraid of what people would think if they knew. If I felt ashamed and disgusted, others had to feel the same way.

This extended to dating, yet another prospect fraught with anxiety. Tearfully, I asked my closest friend Nancy, "How can I possibly share this with a man, and how will he understand?"

She listened and tried to console me. "Guys are different," she said gently. "They really don't care about that."

I didn't believe her, but I knew she was trying very hard to make me feel better. I agreed to a few dates, but fearing humiliation and rejection if I shared my secret, I never made promises to further the relationship.

The walls of my world gradually closed in until the bathroom became both my refuge and my prison.

CHAPTER 8

Who Knew Seattle Had Hills?

I'd been living in Denver since 1971, and by the late 1970s, the city had started to lose its appeal. Over the years, I watched as urban sprawl and the dreaded "brown cloud" of smog changed the character and odor of the city I'd been in love with. The air, no longer pristine and pure, smelled foul, and the Rocky Mountains—those solid, majestic peaks capped with sparkling snow—were no longer visible on days when the pollution was heavy.

One morning, I sat bolt upright in bed and knew I was really ready to leave the Mile-High City. But I had no desire to go back to Pittsburgh, the accents in the South would grate on my nerves, there was nothing that interested me in the Midwest, and I wasn't fond of the great state of California.

The Pacific Northwest, however, seemed romantic, with its soft blanket of fog hiding tall evergreen trees, water, and ferryboats. Despite my friends' warnings of constant rain, I was not deterred.

I left Colorado on a clear October day in 1979. My AAA map and the name of the one person I could call once I got there were on the dashboard of my Datsun B-210. I packed my car with my clothes, some cooking utensils, my little stereo, and a couple of pictures. The rest of my worldly possessions were stored at a friend's house.

Three days later, I arrived in Seattle. I could smell the moisture in the air, and feel it on my skin.

I'd grown so accustomed to the dry, mile-high air that I felt as if I'd had a series of collagen injections. *Wow*, I thought. *What a great way to take five years off my face!*

I set my destination to the YWCA. I figured I'd find my way by following the signs toward the city center, which brought me to the downtown area. One of the first things I noticed were the hills. As I headed up Spring Street, I fervently prayed that I would make the light at the crest of the hill. "Please, God, please let me make this light. I'll observe the Sabbath, I'll go to services every Friday night and Saturday, I'll keep Kosher. I'll . . ." I did not make the light. My car, tuned for high altitude, was now at sea level, and the carburetor protested loudly. I didn't have a clue how to operate a stick shift while stopped on a hill. There were no hills in Denver, and I started to wonder why I had left.

The light turned green. My foot came off the brake and clutch, but before I could depress the gas pedal, the car stalled and rolled back. I sat through two light changes, repeating this process. My heart pounded, and I nervously glanced in the rearview mirror, expecting the drivers to begin a noisy horn tirade. It didn't happen. Just silence.

A wave of relief swept over me when a police officer riding a motorcycle came to my rescue. He stared at me through his mirrored, aviator sunglasses. His chiseled facial features and thin mouth barely moved as he asked what my problem was. I patiently explained the situation, adding, "I'm from Denver," in the hopes that it would elicit sympathy. He continued to stare.

With a short blast on his whistle, I was directed to back onto a level area next to the sidewalk and start the car again. The carburetor roared back to life.

The officer sneered. "If I hold the traffic, can you get your car up the rest of the hill?" he asked. My answer was to floor the gas pedal, and I shot up the hill.

The YWCA had no vacant rooms, so the staff directed me to the Kennedy Hotel. I woke the following morning and looked out the window to a world enveloped in fog. Ferryboat fog horns blared, and I inhaled the salty air. Anxious to explore, I got in touch with my only contact in the area. Charlie came over and took me on a tour of the city, ending down at the waterfront, where he introduced me to fresh Penn Cove mussels.

With his help, I secured an apartment in the same large, brick building he lived in. It was being renovated, and the landlord promised I'd be upgraded to the next new unit. The area looked a bit seedy, but the bright side was that it was located across the street from a prison work-release program, so the police had a strong presence in the neighborhood. *It's temporary*, I told myself. Small, dead bugs (that I convinced myself were just caraway seeds) littered the unit, but I needed to save money, and I couldn't afford to stay in the hotel.

In between tracking down job leads and registering with temporary secretarial agencies, my biggest task would be to master driving my stick shift on Seattle's daunting hills. My first method was avoidance. I would think, *Can I get to where I need to go without encountering a hill?* When it was apparent that this wouldn't be possible, I remembered my father saying, "Lois, you can do anything you put your mind to." With determination, I mastered driving on Seattle's hills in six weeks!

I had a series of apartments in a couple of different neighborhoods, took on a variety of jobs, and learned to love hearing the sound of rain from the time I woke up to the time I went to bed. I appreciated the spectacular sunsets both in winter and summer, made even more beautiful when filtered through clouds. My breath caught in my throat when I saw the majestic beauty of Mt. Rainier, especially in the winter, when natives would say, "The mountain is out." Feeling the spray of water on my face while on a ferryboat, and hearing the seagulls as they circled overhead, brought a smile to my face. I loved the excitement of shopping for food at the Pike Place Market, and the bustle of the crowds. I marveled at how long daylight lasted during the summer. I even loved the clouds as I discerned different patterns and shades of gray.

Over the course of five years, Crohn's disease lurked, slowly tunneling through my colon and leaving scar tissue in its wake. Incidents of increasing bowel incontinence, fevers, extreme fatigue, diarrhea, and weight loss increased, signaling that the disease was growing stronger. Steroids kept the disease corralled, though eventually I had to be hospitalized for short periods of time. Then, severe diarrhea sent me into acidosis shock that resulted in another hospital stay. I was desperate to try anything, even acupuncture, to slow the progression of the disease. Colonoscopies revealed what I didn't want to admit: my entire colon and rectum were diseased.

In 1984, I found myself sitting on the exam table in my doctor's office, hearing the words I'd been terrified of since my initial diagnosis when I was a sick and frightened seventeen-year-old.

CHAPTER 9

Confronting Ostomy Surgery

I was always afraid of having a colostomy. I didn't really know what the surgery entailed, only that it should be avoided. When diagnosed with Crohn's disease, I asked every doctor, "Will I have to get a colostomy?" They all answered no. Why tell a teenage girl that ostomy surgery might be in her future?

The procedure is still misunderstood, much the same way mastectomy surgery for those with breast cancer was forty years ago. It's time for ostomy surgery to come out of the bathroom and into the living room.

"We can't keep taking sections out of your gut and suturing you back together," my doctor said. "It's time to discuss ostomy surgery." I was thirty-four.

I reacted with panic and terror. "No, you aren't going to mutilate me," I said. Then I ran out of his office, tears streaming down my face and blurring my vision.

But more bowel resections were no longer an option. I had to consider undergoing a total procto-colectomy (removal of my colon and rectum) and permanent ileostomy (rerouting of the small bowel through the abdominal wall, allowing drainage of intestinal matter into an external "ostomy pouching system" located on my lower-right abdomen).

I spent the next two years fighting a battle I could not win. I was constantly exhausted, and I never weighed much more than ninety pounds. After a routine colonoscopy, the doctor stood at the foot of the bed and said, "Lois, the last time you had this exam, you had two strictures in your colon. This time, you have double that amount. The handwriting is on the wall." His words pierced through the cushion of drugs I'd received prior to the procedure, and I felt my stomach lurch.

Later that day, I called my doctor and informed him I'd made the decision to have ostomy surgery. I shared the news with my parents, but I didn't want anyone else in the family to know about my decision. I was fearful of how I would be seen, and I didn't have the fortitude to handle what I thought would be pitying looks and whispered comments about "having the bag."

Ostomy surgery meant facing my nightmare head on, and fear spread its tentacles, trying to convince me to change my mind. My doctor wisely knew that I needed to talk to someone who was living with an ileostomy. He gave me the name of a woman close to my age who'd also needed an ostomy because of Crohn's disease. "The two of you should meet," he told me. "You need to talk with her." This was 1986, before HIPAA dictated patient privacy rules.

After a brief talk with my new "ostomy mentor," we made arrangements to meet at a local restaurant. Like an Olympic athlete, I went into training to prepare for this rendezvous. The day before the meeting I ate only sparingly, and the morning of, I only had small amounts of water, and prescription-strength medication to control diarrhea.

I arrived early and selected a table where I could see who walked in but still had some privacy. Suddenly, a tall, stunning woman wearing a skintight jumpsuit came in, smiled, and introduced herself. I'd been openly staring, my eyes scanning her abdominal area. My mother's voice in my head said, *"Lois, it's not polite to stare."* I nearly muttered, "Not now, Ma, I'm busy." One thought played over and over in my mind. *Where's the bag hidden?*

Myth number one about ostomy surgery: you can only wear baggy, shapeless clothes. I was relieved. I could still shop at Nordstrom's.

She encouraged me to ask anything about her surgery, even if I thought it was too personal. The questions tumbled out of my mouth, coming fast and furious. What was it like having a bowel movement through a stoma? What about intimacy? Would anyone know I had an ostomy? Would I smell? In between questions, I sprinted to the bathroom. But not my mentor. I was secretly impressed. Maybe there were some advantages to ostomy surgery after all.

Two hours later, she asked me why I wanted to have the surgery. I gave her the usual answers of being tired of having bowel incontinence and always needing to know the location of a bathroom. She looked at me intently. "I have an assignment for you," she said. "I want you to list everything you hate about having Crohn's disease. I think this exercise will help you with your decision." We picked a date to get together at her home in a few days, and she gave me some pouching-system samples.

Once home, I shoved the samples under the bed. I wasn't ready to imagine what I would look like with one adhered to my abdomen. After reviewing the day's events, I was ready to tackle my "homework." I came up with fifteen reasons why I hated having Crohn's disease.

When I finished writing "I'm tired of being an observer of life and not an active participant," I put the pen down, staring at what I'd written. Something shifted in that moment; I could no longer deny how narrow and constricted my life had become. Over the years, I'd changed my life to accommodate a disease that wanted to keep me confined to a bathroom, had destroyed my self-confidence, and had scarred me both internally and externally.

I realized that I was now emotionally ready to go forward with ostomy surgery. I was still scared, but I instinctively knew that I was headed in the direction of living my life instead of being a passive observer.

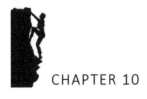

CHAPTER 10

Stoma 101

When the small or large bowel is brought up through the abdominal wall and adhered with sutures, the part of the bowel that remains above the skin is called a stoma.

Stoma is a Greek word meaning mouth or new opening. Ostomy surgery diverts stool or urine from its normal evacuation route to this new opening. Ostomy surgery crosses all age groups, and can be necessary because of colorectal cancer, inflammatory bowel disease (IBD), bladder cancer, or trauma to the gut, such as a gunshot wound.

At the time that I was learning about this surgery, I was unaware that a national organization existed for people with ostomies: the United Ostomy Associations of America (UOAA). Formerly known as the United Ostomy Association (UOA), the UOAA provides education and assistance to those undergoing ostomy surgery, as well as their family members and friends. The UOAA estimates that there are approximately 750,000 individuals in the United States living with an ostomy.

The next meeting with my ostomy mentor was at her home. There, I came face to face with a stoma. Up until that time, I'd only seen photographs of what I would soon have on my own abdomen. It was time to go further, and get up close and personal with a part of my body that normally didn't see the light of day.

The UOA had a training course for individuals

who had gone through ostomy surgery themselves, so they could visit with and mentor people who were planning for or had already had the surgery.

What my mentor showed me that day was definitely not UOA-approved protocol, but it was incredibly helpful and enlightening. I listened as she explained what I would see firsthand: her taking off the pouching system covering her stoma and applying a new one. My heart began beating faster, and a wave of anxiety washed over me. I felt the familiar movement in my abdomen indicating the need to get to a bathroom quickly or risk an accident. Feeling the blood plummet to my feet, I blurted out a quick apology and rushed headlong into the place that offered temporary refuge. It took a few minutes for the pounding in my chest to subside and the roiling in my gut to slow down.

Once I saw her stoma, the anxiety and fear vanished, replaced with wonder. I saw part of her small bowel, and watched the peristaltic motion of the GI tract as it contracted and elongated. I also learned that the bright-red color was an indication of a healthy bowel.

Utterly fascinated, I looked at my mentor. "That's what a stoma looks like? That's what I'll have? I can handle that." After a few more seconds of eye contact, I laughingly said, "It almost looks like a small penis!" No offense to any men reading this, and of course, I knew the difference between the two. My comment was the humor I needed to break the chain of fear that had held me prisoner whenever I thought about living without a colon.

I intently watched as my mentor cleaned the skin around the stoma (known as peristomal skin), and then explained each step as she put on a new pouching system. I learned the difference between changing a pouching system and emptying its contents. Ideally, three to five days was the optimal wear time between system changes. Emptying would depend on what food and how much of it I consumed, and whether it was low or high in fiber.

With an ileostomy, the remaining small bowel slowly "learns" to take on the function of the colon, which mainly reabsorbs water into the body. Right after surgery, my output would be mostly liquid, but over time, it would become more formed and semi-solid.

I kept in regular contact with my mentor, and slowly, the idea of having an ileostomy was not as daunting and frightening as it had been prior to our first meeting. That didn't mean I totally embraced my decision to have the surgery, however.

Fear and myths surround ostomy surgery. We often use phrases like "go with your gut," "trust your gut instinct," or "she has guts," but when it actually comes to talking about that part of our body, we're reluctant to admit that we all poop. When guts go awry, we exhibit the "turtle syndrome": we retreat inwardly, laugh nervously, and put our hands over our ears and eyes.

The media has also been slow to educate the public about ostomy surgery; up until recently, it received little coverage. Comedians have used the tired line, "Ostomy surgery isn't so bad, except I have trouble finding shoes to match my bag." Medical television shows have covered a wide variety of procedures with great empathy, but not ostomy surgery. Harsh comments from TV surgeons and doctors such as "really, how do you sugarcoat a colostomy bag?" and "we'll see about getting rid of the poo bag for you" only serve to perpetuate fears and myths about this life-saving and life-giving surgical procedure.

It's time to confront the myths that you'll smell, that everyone will know, that you'll be confined to your home, and that you'll be living on the sidelines. These fears made me keep a death grip on my colon and rectum long after it was evident that how I was managing my Crohn's disease was no longer effective. Even after I realized that I had no quality of life and made the decision to go ahead with ostomy surgery, I emphatically told my parents that no one else in the family could know about my decision.

I soon met another woman who'd had an ileostomy, hers due to ulcerative colitis. Just like my ostomy mentor, she was healthy, active, and completely comfortable with her ostomy. If she hadn't told me about her surgery, I never would have known. The more time I spent with these two women, the more comfortable I became. They were my "bookends" and my role models. If they could triumph and thrive after ostomy surgery, so would I. They provided the courage, confidence, and conviction I needed to go ahead with my decision.

A few days before surgery, I met the Certified Wound, Ostomy, and Continence Nurse (CWOCN®) who would mark the site where the surgeon would pull part of my small bowel through my abdomen. She'd also be my primary nurse after the surgery, teaching me how to care for my stoma, determining the best pouching system for my body's needs, and making herself available when issues arose. She also gave me an additional dose of self-confidence that I would be able to have a full, active life after ostomy surgery. She became the third side to my triangle of resolve.

She guided me through a routine of sitting, standing, and bending from side to side as she observed my body. She explained that this was necessary for good stoma placement. Because I was thin, there was little chance that the stoma would be hidden between folds of skin, but we didn't know how much weight I would gain post-surgery. Normally with an ileostomy, the stoma placement is on the right side of the abdomen. Because of scar tissue from my previous bowel resections, the surgeon felt that my stoma should be on the left side. Scar tissue is different from normal skin, and the pouching system might not adhere as well, compromising the amount of time between pouching system changes. At the end of my visit, I looked down at the X that marked the area where the surgeon would suture the stoma to my abdomen. There was no denying that I was getting closer to the day when the front part of my body would look very different. As if my colon knew what was on the horizon, it lurched violently, and I dashed for the nearest bathroom, releasing a torrent of diarrhea.

The time between my decision to have ostomy surgery and the night before the surgery was only a few weeks. My confidence, however, remained shaky. I still had to conquer the hurdle of that final night.

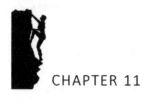

CHAPTER 11

The Night before Ostomy Surgery

We all face "Mount Everest" moments. While they may not come with any media fanfare, these experiences can bring about change in ourselves that is just as satisfying as scaling the world's highest peak.

I was certainly feeling the weight of my own Mount Everest moment the night before my ostomy surgery, when it was time to check into the hospital. After the usual procedures were followed and I'd signed a stack of papers that had surely decimated a small grove of trees, I walked into the hospital room, small suitcase in hand, and surveyed my surroundings. It looked like any hospital room: a bed with handrails in the down position, a little nightstand, a lounging chair, and a television mounted on the wall. The call button for the nurses was clipped to the bedsheet. The curtain on the sealed window fluttered ever so slightly from the circulated air. The bathroom was off to the side.

My parents were with me as I checked in. I knew they were worried, but as much as they wanted to stay with me, I needed to be alone with my thoughts. I told them I loved them, thanked them for their unending support, hugged them tightly, and slowly closed the door as they left.

Silence. I slowly unpacked the few things I'd brought with me and hung my clothes in the narrow closet. *The next time I wear them, I won't have a colon or rectum*, I thought. What would that feel like? I put on the shapeless hospital gown and mismatched bathrobe and climbed into the bed, sliding my feet between the sheets and blanket.

A nurse came in and took my blood pressure, pulse, and temperature. A short time after that, the surgeon arrived. We spoke about my surgery, what he would be doing, and approximately how long he thought the operation would last. "If something goes wrong tomorrow, I don't want to end up being a vegetable," I told him, tears in my eyes.

He looked at me for several moments and then asked what movie I'd watched the night before! He listened to my answer, and then asked me if I had faith in him and his abilities. I nodded, not trusting myself to speak. "What is your religious affiliation?" he asked. I told him I was Jewish. "An ancient and beautiful religion," he said. "With your strong belief and my skill, I promise you will be healthy." He squeezed my hand tightly. "I'll see you tomorrow."

I sat motionless for a long time. Then I slowly swung my feet over the bed and walked to the bathroom. I disrobed and stared at my body in the mirror. The scars from my previous bowel surgeries were clearly visible, even after twenty years. They evidenced the battle I'd fought against Crohn's disease. In spite of the removal of diseased portions of my colon and small bowel and the pharmacological management available at the time, it was a battle that could not be won. If I wanted a chance to be healthy, I had to be willing to give up the diseased parts of my body that Crohn's disease had laid claim to: my colon and rectum.

"Take a good, long look," I said to my reflection. "Starting tomorrow, the front part of your abdomen will look much different."

I panicked. Luckily, I'd brought the piece of paper listing all the reasons I hated Crohn's disease. Frantically, I pawed through my purse, grabbed the creased stationary, and reread my words. Gradually, my hands stopped shaking. My heart slowed to a more normal pace. Folding the paper in half, I went back into the bathroom, took one final look at my bare abdomen and the "X" where the stoma would be, looked into the mirror and said, "I'm ready."

I slept very little that night. Not because I was scared or nervous about my upcoming surgery, but because I was on the phone with one of my ostomy mentors, talking, laughing, and being totally silly and relaxed. When my head finally made contact with the pillow, I was at peace with my decision.

Early the following morning, two nurses transferred me from my bed to a gurney. Yesterday's fear was a dim memory, replaced instead with optimism and confidence. "I'm ready to start living my life," I told them. "Let's get going!"

After I was wheeled into the bright, cold operating room, I watched a team of nurses clothed in green gowns bustle around. The room even smelled cold. Transferred from the gurney onto the operating table, I shivered. I felt a flicker of fear beginning to thread its way through me. Someone put a heated blanket over me, and I relaxed immediately. I looked up and saw my surgeon, mask covering his mouth and a cap over his head. His eyes were warm and reassuring. My arm was taken from under the covers, extended horizontally and taped. The anesthesiologist spoke through his mask, saying I'd soon be getting medication to help me relax. I watched as the rubber tourniquet was tightened around my right bicep, stared as the slender, silver needle entered my vein, and felt a slight burn as the needle delivered the muscle-relaxing medication. My body felt heavy, as if

I was sinking through the table. A whirling sensation created distance between myself and everyone in the room, and voices became faint as I sped toward darkening motionlessness.

I woke to the sound of my name being called. I had a metallic taste in my mouth. The voices sounded far away, but I could feel someone touching me. "You're in the recovery room," someone said. "Your surgery is over. How do you feel?" I suddenly became aware of fiery pain radiating out from my abdomen. "Hurt," escaped from my mouth. An instant later, the relief of oblivion.

When consciousness returned, I was back in my hospital room. My father leaned close to me and asked how I felt. "I feel like a Mack truck ran over me and then backed up and did it again." He squeezed my hand and told me he loved me. My mom did the same. Pain and reality receded as the intravenous opioids coursed through my system. Time ceased to have meaning.

I became conscious of sitting on the edge of the bed, my nurse at my side. The words "we're going to have you sit in the chair" seemed to come from a distance. I have no memory of actually doing that, or of getting back to the soft comfort of the bed and once again escaping to healing sleep.

The following morning, I became more aware of my surroundings. I cautiously pushed the sheets down and pulled my gown up. I wanted to see my stoma. Inside the clear, surgical ostomy pouch, it looked like a large, flattened mushroom. The reality-numbing properties of the drugs circulating through my system kept any fear or anxiety from taking hold.

Later in the day, the surgeon arrived, examined me, and told me about the surgery. "Your colon was literally gray in color," he said. "I have no idea how it could have functioned." The statement floated in the air above my head. "Your stoma looks good," he continued. "It will take another day or so for it to begin functioning. It needs to wake up." I wondered aloud if I would know when that happened. "Believe me, you'll know," he said. Then he patted my shoulder, saying he'd see me the next day.

The routine for the day consisted of sleeping, sitting up in bed, then graduating to an upright chair for a short time. Meals were salty chicken broth.

By the morning of the third day, strange dreams in vivid Technicolor tumbled through my head. Intense movement in my abdomen woke me up. Then it happened again. Had some alien life form found its way inside my body while I lay on the operating room table? I recalled being told that I would know when my stoma and remaining small bowel would "wake up." *Progress*, I thought.

As painful as it was recovering from the procto-colectomy and ileostomy, my body felt the positive difference after only three days. No longer having the diseased and non-functioning large bowel that sapped my energy, I felt stronger and healthier.

By now, the clear pouch had also filled with liquid, which pleased both my nurse and surgeon. Today was the day I would begin walking farther than the distance from the bed to the chair, and I was excited. With a nurse on either side of me, I took several halting steps toward the bathroom, conscious of the weight of the pouch and its movement.

Suddenly, the pouching system pulled away from my skin and fell to the floor, spilling its liquid contents everywhere. I was horrified and deeply ashamed. *I went through surgery for this to happen?* I thought. *Give me back the Crohn's and my non-functioning colon. At least I understood and could deal with that unpredictability.* I instinctively knelt down, frantically trying to figure out how I could clean up the rapidly spreading liquid.

The nurses calmly reassured me that I had on a surgical pouching system that wasn't meant to adhere for more than a few days. Once I had a different system, this wouldn't happen. I felt a little better after hearing their words, but the burning shame and embarrassment would not be consoled so easily. They guided me back to bed, and I watched as one of the ostomy nurses quickly and easily fit me with a more permanent pouching system. My stoma didn't resemble a flattened mushroom, but it still looked large and swollen. I was told it would gradually begin shrinking in size.

After twenty-four hours of tolerating liquids, I happily graduated to a soft diet. I was conscious of food as it moved through my remaining bowel. I started walking around my room, and gradually progressed to the hallway. When I completed one lap, I felt exhausted. I must have looked pretty funny as I walked slowly, one hand pushing the IV pole I'd named Irving, the other pressed against my abdomen. The staples running the length of my stomach made walking upright difficult, so my gait resembled that of an elderly woman.

As my forays into the hospital hallway became longer, I became more conscious of the pouch moving from side to side as I walked. Underwear my mom brought me helped somewhat, and I decided I'd deal with one issue at a time. I bid adieu to Irving, my IV pole, once it became clear that I could tolerate solid food and my stoma was functioning, though at times, it was quite "talkative."

The next hurdle involved having the staples removed. This greatly improved my mobility—I could walk upright and cruise the hospital hallways at speeds I'm sure were well over the legal limit!

My first shower after the surgery was sobering. I let the warm water run over my body, enjoying how it felt on my skin. When I looked down, there was no denying that the clear, plastic pouch was here to stay. I let the tears fall, mingling with the warm water as I finally grieved the colon I'd lost. Strangely, the grief didn't last long. I already felt stronger and more alive, though it had barely been a week since the surgery.

I had a final practice session with one of the hospital's ostomy nurses. Obsessed with knowing everything about the process of taking off a used pouching system and putting on a new one, I kept asking, "Am I doing this right?" She gently assured me I was doing fine, and that in a few weeks, I would be a professional. Knowing I could come in for a consultation if issues arose helped ease my doubts that I wasn't ready to go home and deal with my new way of having a bowel movement. Additionally, my two ostomy mentors were there for me, offering emotional support and technical assistance.

Doctors discharged me after eight days—a length of stay unheard of today. I had a two-week supply of pouching systems, which included wafers, pouches, small scissors, and other needed equipment, along with the name of a medical supply company so I could order additional supplies.

Thanks to an intrepid stoma that I'd nicknamed my "sidekick," I was ready to begin living my life free from Crohn's disease. After twenty years of living with a chronic disease, I was about to find out how wonderful life would be now that I was healthy.

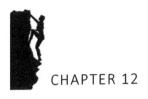

CHAPTER 12

Freedom from Fear

When the majority of your life has been focused on needing to know the exact location of a bathroom, and the fear of not finding it in time, not having to do that anymore is exhilarating.

Arriving home from the hospital after my ostomy surgery was a time filled with excitement and some fear. While it felt good to be home, I still struggled with nervousness about caring for my ostomy by myself. I was also very gut-focused. Every abdominal sound was magnified, and I could feel food traversing through my remaining small intestine. I still ate a low-residue diet, so salads, fresh fruit, and foods high in fiber were still off-limits. My output consistency was still mostly liquid, and I noticed the warmth of the contents throughout the day.

When the time came to change the pouching system and apply a new one, I was nervous. Would I do it right? Should I call one of my ostomy mentors to come over for support?

My mom also expressed interest in watching. Her support and willingness to learn was overwhelming and greatly appreciated. Her confidence in my ability to master post-ostomy care gave me the courage I needed, and I found myself in the role of a teacher again.

I laid out all my supplies on the bathroom counter: wafer, pouch, scissors, stoma measuring guide, adhesive remover towelette, skin barrier towelette, barrier ring, washcloth, and toilet paper. After carefully removing the old pouching system with the adhesive remover towelette, I gently patted the skin around the stoma with the washcloth and allowed it to dry. Using the stoma measuring guide, I could see how much my stoma had come down in size. I traced the opening that corresponded to the stoma size onto the back of the wafer, and cut it to match the size of my stoma.

I explained each step in the process to my mom and felt my self-confidence in managing my stoma increase. I applied the protective skin barrier towelette around the stoma, and after it was dry, I placed the protective barrier ring over it, and then finally the wafer. The final step was to snap the pouch onto the wafer. I turned to my mom and said, " Piece of cake!" We hugged. Gratitude for my mother's support welled up, and tears rolled down my face as we hugged and laughed.

My confidence increased with every pouching change, but it was reassuring to know that I could call my mentors or the ostomy nurse at the out-patient clinic if any issues arose.

Soon, the day came to venture out of the safety of my parent's home and back into the real world. My father was planning a surprise party to honor his and my mom's upcoming anniversary, and he wanted my help in picking out a card. When we arrived at the card store, old behavior patterns that had deeply burrowed into my brain reared up, and I tried to search out the public restroom in case the need arose. I scanned the store's landscape, then realized that this behavior was no longer necessary. It took a few minutes for this understanding to sink in. When it did, the freedom I felt nearly overwhelmed me. A small grin appeared at the corners of my mouth and then widened into a full-fledged smile. My entire body seemed to breathe a sigh of relief.

I experienced freedom for the first time in twenty years: freedom from having to know the exact location of a bathroom; freedom from bowel incontinence; freedom to walk in the park, watch a movie, or enjoy a meal without running to the bathroom; freedom to really listen to someone while they spoke instead of worrying if my body would betray or embarrass me.

Now that I grew more comfortable with my ostomy, I was anxious to try those activities I'd been fearful of doing in the past. Could I really sit through an entire movie without running to the bathroom? What better test than to see *Aliens*! I sat through the entire movie and didn't miss any of the high points, including when the queen alien is threatening the young girl, Newt, and Sigourney Weaver yells, "Get away from her, you bitch!" and then proceeds to kill the queen and her eggs in an epic battle.

Once the surgeon and gastroenterologist formally discharged me, the time came to move back to Seattle. What would life be like now that I was no longer burdened with a diseased colon and rectum?

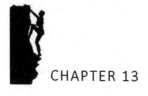

CHAPTER 13

New Adventures in Seattle

To say my life took a 180-degree turn for the better after ostomy surgery would be an understatement. It wasn't all smooth sailing; I still faced challenges, and I had obstacles to climb and lessons to learn. But at least I was healthy, and that made all the difference for me.

One of my mother's favorite expressions was, "If you have your health, you have everything." Her other inspiring expressions, along with my father's supportive words from so long ago, echoed in my mind as I returned to Seattle in the fall of 1986. It felt good to be home. My friends Lynn and Jeff offered to let me stay with them until I found a job and saved up the money for a place of my own.

My first job post-surgery ended up being in a gourmet deli in Pike Place Market. I'd always loved the Market, as Seattleites call it, and working there brought back memories of my parents' grocery store in Pittsburgh. The sights, sounds, and smells of the Market energized me. There was a force there that felt almost electric, and I loved it. The deli attracted a variety of people and the hours seemed to fly by.

My fear that I wouldn't like myself after surgery never became a reality, and even though I was very willing to share details about my surgery with my friends, I was finding out how much and who to share this information with. I wasn't going around intro-ducing everyone to my "sidekick" or showing off my battle scars, but I was learning that not everyone wanted to know all the details about my surgery. Some did, but others were just happy that I was healthy and said, "No details, please."

One day, after being at work for about an hour, I thought I felt wetness around the area of my stoma. It's one thing to experience this in the comfort of your home, but at work, it brings out a new level of anxiety. I told my coworker and manager I needed a bathroom break. My heart pounded as I envisioned the seal around the wafer being compromised. A wave of relief washed over me when I realized my pouching system was secure and what I'd felt was normal output. Because my ostomy was so recent, the output was still watery.

I made a decision to share a brief overview of my surgery with my coworker. Would she view me differently? Would I see compassion and empathy in her eyes, or something else? Hesitantly, I shared a little about my life with Crohn's disease and my recent ostomy surgery. I held my breath after I finished, scanning her face for any sign of disgust. Instead, she thanked me for letting her know that there would be times I'd need access to the bathroom more often than the rest of my coworkers. She said she was happy that I was now healthy. If it would've been appropriate, I would have hugged her. Instead, I thanked her for her understanding.

As much fun as it was working at the Market, I knew I needed a job with better pay and benefits. I applied for a position with a local commercial real-estate firm, and landed it.

A few hours into my first day, my boss came out of his office and told me that the last call I'd answered was from his wife. She had apparently told him, "Charlie, I don't know who she is, but make sure you do whatever is necessary to have her stay. Her phone voice is very professional." The work itself wasn't too difficult, but learning how to use the computer was a different matter. My coworker was tasked with teaching me, which turned out to not be my ideal learning environment.

A few months later, I received a call from a reporter for the *Seattle Times*. They were conducting research on individuals who didn't have health insurance, and how that impacted their lives. I responded with my story and was chosen to be part of the article. Even though my current job provided benefits, there was still a waiting period before the health insurance would be active, and it excluded any pre-existing conditions. Anything related to my ostomy surgery would not be covered. About fifteen minutes into the face-to-face interview, I felt wetness through my skirt and realized that the seal on my wafer had become compromised. Trying to concentrate on the reporter's questions and appear calm took every ounce of resolve I had. The photographer told me to look distressed for the picture, which was no problem! I only had to keep my hand inside my skirt pocket to feel the spreading wetness over my abdomen.

After the interview, which took place at work, I told Charlie I needed to go home. He gave me a puzzled look. I still didn't know him very well, so I said, "I have a situation I need to take care of at home. Imagine that I have to change a tire, but instead, it has to do with surgery I recently had on my digestive tract." He told me to go home and deal with whatever had to be done, no explanation necessary. I was grateful for his understanding.

Very early one morning, I woke up with a severe case of uncontrolled diarrhea. A little later, I knew something was wrong. My head felt heavy and I was having difficulty concentrating. I knew I needed to get to the emergency room. I called Charlie, who rushed over and got me to the Harborview Medical Center. Doctors started me on an IV and drew blood for testing. Twenty minutes later, my cubicle in the hospital was buzzing with activity. I heard, "Change that IV, stat. Elevated potassium."

One of the adverse consequences of diarrhea is depleted potassium, a necessary electrolyte. I had been on a medication to help raise my potassium levels, but I didn't realize that there might be consequences to not being monitored while on the supplement. In the ER, nurses changed the IV bag, stuck electrodes on my body for an EKG, and whisked me to the intensive care unit. Anxious faces of the nursing staff stared at me, asking if I felt all right. I was discharged later that day, after my potassium fell within normal range. The only explanation given was that because the diarrhea was so severe, it had caused the increased potassium to become very concentrated and rise to a critical level.

After several months, it became obvious that I wasn't happy at my job, and that continuing to stay was counterproductive. The parting was cordial. I secured a temporary position in the development office of the Fred Hutchinson Cancer Research Center, where I processed and acknowledged contributions to the center.

Working a variety of temporary positions had lost its appeal. While on my way to drop off some resumes one day, I tripped on the sidewalk. As I went sailing through the air I was surprised that I'd tripped, because I didn't recall seeing anything out of the ordinary. Not wanting to injure my stoma, I turned in midair to avoid my left side and landed squarely on my right hip, arms outstretched. My purse landed a few feet away from me. I yelled for help, and a passerby phoned an ambulance while someone else retrieved my purse and scattered paperwork.

The paramedics arrived a short time later. When I tried to stand, my leg buckled. Pain radiated from my right groin. "I think you have a muscle injury," the medic said. "Just take pain medication and stay off of it for a while."

Another medic came over, and by this time, I was starting to go into shock. I trembled uncontrollably. They placed a blanket over my shoulders. "See if you can stand up," the second emergency tech said. My leg wouldn't support my weight, and the pain was intensifying. The tech said, "I think you have a break. We need to get you to Harborview."

The enormity of the situation started to sink in. Because I was working as a temp, I didn't have health insurance. How could I afford the ambulance ride, or a visit to the ER? I made the medics put me in the passenger seat of my car, and a friend who owned a business a block away came and drove me to the trauma center. As I sat in my car, I wondered what the next step would be.

It seemed to take forever to be seen. I wasn't visibly bleeding, so my condition wasn't seen as critical, despite the mounting pain. When I was finally wheeled into an examination room, I felt a little better. At least I would get some answers. Just as a resident began to examine me, I heard someone being wheeled into the adjacent examination room. Someone said, "Eyes fixed and dilated." I'd watched enough medical dramas on TV to know this wasn't a good sign. The resident rushed over and the drape was quickly pulled shut, but I could still hear the conversation and knew at a gut level that this individual was likely terminal.

When I was finally examined, the resident explained that I had likely sustained a hip fracture. A fracture didn't sound as bad to me as "broken," and I shared this with the doctor. He looked at me and then carefully and slowly explained that "fracture" and "broken" are the same thing. My remaining guts twisted inside. "We'll know the exact location and extent of the injury after we see the x-rays, so let's get you down there," the resident said. I was scheduled for surgery in the morning.

Two days later, after receiving training on how to use crutches, I was discharged. My compromised mobility lasted three months. It was challenging, but I survived. Changing my pouching system while standing on one leg was tiring at first, but over time, my good leg became stronger.

Three months of limited mobility afforded me time to think and reflect. I was no longer afraid to talk about my life with active Crohn's disease. I knew, however, that many people were uncomfortable discussing anything related to their digestive system. Medical shows on TV dealt with many diseases, but none of them ever mentioned Crohn's disease, ulcerative colitis, or ostomy surgery. I found myself getting angry. Why weren't we discussing digestive diseases?

I decided it was long overdue to have a frank, honest discussion about IBD, the umbrella term used to describe Crohn's disease, ulcerative colitis, and ostomy surgery, on the talk shows that were popular in the late 1980s. After watching all of them, I decided to contact the *Sally Jessy Raphael Show*. Miraculously, I actually reached a producer, something unheard of today. I'd rehearsed a speech and written down some key points I wanted to discuss.

Alex, the producer, was unimpressed. He told me he had no intentions of doing a show about diarrhea. I agreed and said that I had no interest in watching an hour-long show about loose bowel movements, but the topic still needed attention. Undaunted and determined, I persisted. For every one of Alex's objections, I had a comeback. The tide began turning when we discussed health insurance coverage, or the lack thereof due to pre-existing conditions. Once he heard firsthand what I had gone through, his demeanor shifted.

At the time, there were very few public figures who would admit to having inflammatory bowel disease, let alone to having undergone ostomy surgery. But I knew of a few of them, and once I started mentioning their names, I could almost hear Alex's thoughts of rising ratings for the show. "If you can guarantee that they'll appear on the show, I'll do it," he said. I had confidence they would, but told him I'd have to check with them first just in case. Victory definitely tasted sweet!

I already knew that Rolf Benirschke (former placekicker for the San Diego Chargers), Marvin Bush (brother of George W. Bush), and Mary Ann Mobley (actress and former Miss America) had been contacted by the National Foundation for Ileitis and Colitis (NFIC), today known as the Crohn's & Colitis Foundation of America (CCFA), and that they had agreed to lend their voices for IBD awareness. I called the communications director for the NFIC at the time, told her the good news, and she handled the remaining details.

In the early summer of 1989, I flew to New York City and was met by a limousine driver who took me to a bed and breakfast in Connecticut. I'd never been in a limousine, and the entire experience was exciting.

The next morning during breakfast, I went over my talking points. *Relax*, I told myself. *You know your own story.* Not knowing the questions I would be asked or how much time I'd have to talk, it was important to be as succinct as possible.

It was a short drive to the studio, where I finally got to meet Alex after months of conversation. Suddenly, I was in the green room. The studio had provided food and refreshments, but I was too nervous and excited to eat. Alex came in and gave me an overview of how the show was arranged and in what order the guests would be featured. The feeling was surreal. I was actually going to be on national television, in front of a live studio audience. A makeup artist came in and fluffed up my hair and made sure I had enough color on my cheeks.

Finally, during the third segment, it was my turn. Alex escorted me to the set. "Just look at Sally and talk to her. You don't have to look at the camera." My heart pounded with excitement, along with a hefty dose of fear! I went into automatic pilot and couldn't tell you exactly what I said. After the first few minutes, I found my stride and my voice. Then it was over, or so I thought. I was back in the green room when I heard I was wanted onstage. Alex introduced me to the audience as being the driving force behind creating an open discussion of IBD— something, he said, would not have happened otherwise. The sound of the applause from the audience was overwhelming and totally unexpected.

After thanking Sally and Alex, I was once again in a limousine being driven to John F. Kennedy International Airport, where I caught my flight home to Seattle. I had to keep telling myself that the entire experience had really happened; it wasn't a dream. Memories came back of the day I received the diagnosis of Crohn's disease, of how frightened and angry I was, and of my father's words when I asked him, "Why me?" Could this experience of sharing my story on national television be what he meant?

Several years later, I sat at my computer, and began writing my story. Words tumbled over each other as I typed. Memories I thought I had dealt with and locked away began to surface. I relived those early years of abdominal pain, rampant diarrhea, severe weight loss, and humiliating incontinence that led to my obsession with knowing the location of every bathroom. I remembered the times when I felt the walls of my world closing in, relegating me to stay a prisoner in my own home. It was then I realized that ostomy surgery had given me back everything that Crohn's disease had taken from me; it had given me back my life. I kept writing until I completed the first draft at around two in the morning. I was working in the English department of the University of Washington at the time, and some of the professors I'd become friends with volunteered to read and edit what I'd written.

My initial thought was to contact magazines in the hopes of getting my story published. About six weeks after mailing the manuscript to a targeted publication, I received my first rejection letter. Attached was a handwritten note that said not to give up. I shared this with the English professors who'd helped, saying, "You know you're a writer when you get your first rejection slip!"

I then thought of Rolf Benirschke and wondered if he might have some ideas for me. I tracked down his email address and contacted him. He called me and explained that he was putting together a book of stories showing that ostomy surgery was not the end of your life, but the beginning. He asked to see my story. Excited, I emailed it to him and heard back a few days later that he wanted to include my story in his book!

Great Comebacks from Ostomy Surgery was published in 2002, and I received several complimentary copies. I was now a published writer! I gave one to my doctor, Deborah Klein, who promptly told me that I needed to share my story with University of Washington medical students. "They need to hear this," she said. "They have a very full curriculum and I don't know how you'll be able to fit this in, but that's your assignment!" When your doctor tells you to do something, you listen and follow through, right?

Several phone calls later, I was able to talk with the instructor who coordinated the gastroenterology portion of the curriculum for the students. He figured out how to fit my talk into their first-year schedule. Those talks paved the way for me to begin speaking to nursing students at the University of Washington and at two other universities in Seattle. Many students told me how my story helped them personalize Crohn's disease, ulcerative colitis, and ostomy surgery. The biggest compliment was when I would hear that, as a result of my talk, a student had decided to either specialize in GI nursing or become a Certified Wound, Ostomy, and Continence Nurse (CWOCN®).

Without my realizing it, I became a patient advocate for the IBD and ostomy community. Once again, I thought of the words my father had said to me so long ago. They had not only proven true, but continued to inspire me.

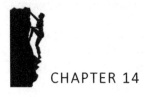

CHAPTER 14

Lois Goes to Washington . . . Olympia, Washington

I firmly believe that some people come into our lives for a reason. It might be to help us make a decision about an important matter, gain insight into ourselves, or inspire us to do something that ultimately helps others. Ally Bain was one of these people.

I met Ally and her mother, Lisa, in January of 2008, at a sales meeting that UCB, a biopharmaceutical company, was having in California.

When Ally was fourteen, she and her mom were shopping in a popular retail store in suburban Chicago when Ally desperately needed to use the bathroom. After several urgent requests that included an explanation of Ally's medical condition, the store manager refused to grant her access to the "employee-only" restroom. As a result, Ally had a humiliating accident. Instead of remaining quiet about this devastating situation, mother and daughter contacted the media, and Ally's experience got the attention of a local television station.

Ally also contacted Kathy Ryg, an Illinois state representative, who helped pass the Restroom Access Act (also known as Ally's Law) in the state in August 2005. The law guaranteed people with certain medical conditions the right to use a bathroom in an emergency, including "employee-designated" bathrooms.

Ally's experience resonated with me. I'd been in similar situations, and having to beg to use a store's bathroom is psychologically devastating and degrading. Ally's courage and determination made an impression.

A month later, I was still thinking about what had happened to this young teen and the resulting legislation in Illinois. Six or seven states had soon passed their own Restroom Access Acts, with legislation pending in many others. Could I get something similar passed in the state of Washington? The thought kept running through my mind.

After staring at the blinking cursor, I composed an email to Marko Liias, my district's state representative, explaining the essence of the bill and why I was so passionate about getting similar legislation enacted in Washington state. I reread what I'd written several times. Suddenly, I heard my mother's voice in my head, intoning one of her favorite expressions, *"Poop or get off the pot, Lois."* I immediately clicked the send button. It's best not to question voices or messages from the great beyond!

On the bus ride home from work, my cell phone rang. Absently, I answered. The voice on the other end identified himself, saying he'd read my email and wanted to talk further about my idea for legislation. I glanced at my watch and thought, *Wow, this guy is still at work and it's after 5:00 p.m.* Still in shock, I asked, "Who are you again?" Laughing, Representative Liias repeated his name and we discussed where the idea for the bill had come from. When asked if I would be willing to testify before House and Senate committee meetings, I agreed. We set a future date for a face-to-face meeting in Olympia, Washington. "This is even better than getting a call from Oprah!" I said. Representative Liias responded with a laugh.

To prepare for this preliminary meeting with the initial committee members, I put together a packet that included information about Crohn's disease and the Restroom Access Act, active and pending state legislation, a list of resources, and an article about how Ally's Law was passed in Illinois.

I'd never made a presentation before elected officials or committee members, but I didn't let that dissuade me. The individuals whom Representative Liias had initially drafted for the committee were enthusiastic and on board with the idea of the proposed legislation. Representative Liias promised to keep me informed, and asked me to think about key individuals who would testify with me when the bill came up for a hearing before the House of Representatives. He cautioned that the political process would not happen overnight, and the bill would be introduced in the 2009 legislative session.

Following the bill's progress during both House and Senate proceedings was an amazing education. I had never been interested in how a bill became law and had no idea about the number of steps proposed legislation goes through. This experience made it personal, and it was exciting, suspenseful, and nerve-racking at the same time.

House Bill 1138 was first read on January 14, 2009 and referred on to Judiciary. I received notice from Representative Liias that the first hearing in the House Committee would be on January 29, and that I would need to be in Olympia to testify alongside two other advocates for the bill, Rob Menaul and Mike McCready, the lead guitarist for Pearl Jam. Knowing I'd have a designated amount of time to talk, I wrote down key points and practiced my speech in front of a mirror.

When the day came, we all met in Representative

Liias's office, were briefed on the proceedings, and went into the House chambers. I had the honor of speaking first. When Rob and Mike concluded, time was allotted for constituent representatives who were opposed to the legislation. An individual representing the restaurant lobby spoke about their concerns. Afterward, he approached Mike and asked him to autograph a Pearl Jam CD! We reconvened in Representative Liias's office to debrief, and the consensus was that the first round had gone well.

A week and a half later, executive action took place, with the first substitute bill being introduced and passed. This meant that some changes had been made to the bill. On February 11, the bill was passed to the Rules Committee for a second reading, and two weeks later, it was on track for another reading by the same committee. On March 3, the substitute bill had a floor amendment, which was adopted and passed on its third reading.

Following along with each step the bill went through felt like a rollercoaster ride. When we received the news of its passage in the House, Rob, Mike, and I were elated. Now it was on to the Senate, where the bill would go through similar steps.

The bill's first reading in the Senate occurred on March 5 and was referred to Judiciary. I received an email from Representative Liias letting me know there would be a public hearing on March 25. He stressed the importance of having additional individuals there to testify on behalf of the bill. I worked with the Pacific Northwest chapter of the Crohn's & Colitis Foundation of America (CCFA), and together we assembled a group of individuals who would accompany me to Olympia to share our stories. Mike McCready once again gave his support and testified.

Two days later, executive action was taken in the Senate. We encountered a brief stumbling block when the retail association wanted extra steps enacted in the bill for safeguards against possible merchandise theft. By the end of March, the bill was passed with the amendment and it was sent to the Rules Committee in the Senate for a second reading. By the middle of April, the bill had proceeded through a second reading by the Rules Committee, and with no further amendments after a third reading, it passed on April 14.

My excitement lasted only four days. The House refused to concur with the changes the Senate had made in committee, and they asked the Senate to recede from the amendments. It was a tense moment—we were so close to having the bill enacted. On April 22, the Senate receded from the amendments, and it passed with a 33-12 vote!

On April 24, the Speaker of the House signed the bill. The following day, the bill was signed by the President of the Senate and delivered to the governor.

The entire process of how a bill gets passed was an eye-opening experience. I was amazed at the number of bills introduced at the start of a legislative session that actually end up passing.

On May 11, I was in Olympia along with Mike McCready, his wife Ashley O'Connor, Barb Wodzin, Rob Menaul, Broh Landsman, Esten Gose, and Jennifer O'Connor. We represented the Pacific Northwest CCFA chapter. Members of Representative Liias's staff also joined us as Governor Christine Gregoire signed the Restroom Access Bill into law for Washington state, with an effective date of July 26, 2009.

On September 16, Linda Huse, the executive director of the CCFA, awarded me with a plaque commending my work on the Restroom Access Bill.

At the CCFA's Northwest chapter luncheon in May of 2010, I received the Mike McCready & Ashley O'Connor Award in recognition for my support of the bill. Representative Marko Liias received an award as well.

I had no way of knowing that meeting a courageous teen and her mother would ultimately motivate me to take action. That was all the inspiration I needed, along with the words, *"Poop or get off the pot, Lois!"*

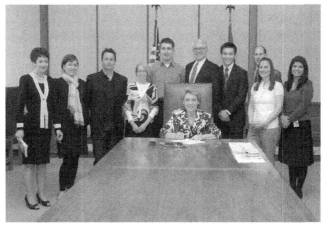

From left: me, Ashley O'Connor, Mike McCready, Barb Wodzin, Esten Gose, Rob Menaul, Kyle Gotchy, Broh Landsman, Jennifer O'Connor, and Jennifer Waldref. Governor Christine Gregoire is seated.

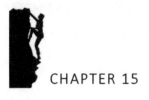

CHAPTER 15

What about Intimacy?

The Beatles' popular song about still being loved at sixty-four wasn't exactly on my mind when I contemplated my ostomy surgery. I was concerned about the immediate future. Would I still be attractive to someone after ostomy surgery? Would intimacy be possible?

A few years after my ostomy surgery, I was in my favorite grocery store with a friend who was visiting from Denver. As a treat, I suggested we have oysters on the half shell. A very good-looking man in the seafood department suggested which bivalves we should get, along with a sturdy oyster knife.

"He's really cute," my friend said. "You should go back later and ask him out." We had a delicious dinner that night and laughingly toasted the handsome individual from the seafood counter.

After my friend left, my mind kept wandering back to her comment. It had been a very long time since I'd asked someone I didn't know very well to join me for dinner. After going back and forth about what to do, I finally decided to take a chance. The worst-case scenario was that he would decline, which wouldn't be the end of the world.

I circled the seafood counter several times, trying to be inconspicuous while hoping to spot him. I'm sure I came off as a suspicious shopper to anyone manning the security cameras. *This is silly,* I said to myself. *Just do it!* I rang the service bell and found myself face to face with the very man I'd come to see. After stammering a few times, I told him how much my friend and I had enjoyed the oysters he recommended, and would he be interested in coming over for dinner?

"Only if you let me bring the fish," he replied and laughed.

Not only did Dan bring the fish, but he also insisted on cooking it as well. We had a wonderful evening, and I remember thinking how his bright-blue eyes were such a contrast to his wavy, dark hair. After several more dates, it became evident that we were both interested in taking the relationship to the next level. I didn't know if my ostomy surgery would be an issue, but I knew I had to bring it up and give him the opportunity to ask me questions. Introducing my stoma to someone in the heat of passion was not the best way to proceed.

After another fun evening with Dan, I told him I needed to share my health history with him, and proceeded to tell him about the Crohn's disease and resulting ostomy surgery. He listened intently, and when I finished, he softly said, "It doesn't matter to me—it doesn't change who you are inside. You won't get rid of me that easily."

Dan and I were together for two years, and my ostomy surgery never posed an issue. There were times when my pouch leaked and I had to wake him up to change the sheets. He was always reassuring and loving.

After my relationship with Dan, and despite the numerous warnings about getting involved with a fellow employee, I later found myself interested in one of my coworkers. We had several fun dates and about a month later, we discussed getting intimate. By this time, I had been on a local afternoon talk show discussing Crohn's disease and ostomy surgery. I thought having Tim watch the tape and then answering his questions would be a good segue into discussing my surgery. We made a date for the following week, and he left my place with the tape in hand.

He seemed distant the next week at work, but I convinced myself that I was imagining it. When he picked me up at my apartment to go to an Italian restaurant we both wanted to try, he was unusually quiet. He barely looked at me during dinner, was reluctant to talk, and didn't want to have any physical contact with me. We barely spoke during the car ride back to my apartment. He handed me the tape, and as I asked him what he had thought of the show, he kept backing away, widening the distance between us. "It was definitely BC," he said.

I looked at him and asked, "What's BC?"

"Before contacts," he replied. "You were wearing glasses at the time." Then he turned and walked out the door.

That was the last date I ever had with Tim. I took my coat off, sat on the couch, and realized that his inability to deal with my surgery was his issue, not mine. We all have something we find difficult to accept in someone else. I was secure within myself, and did not take his rejection personally.

Ostomy surgery doesn't change who you are as a person. You're still the same individual with skills, talents, and abilities, except now, you have a better quality of life, and you're healthy. Ostomy surgery is just a slightly different way of going to the bathroom! When you're secure in who you are and accept yourself, others will be comfortable around you as well. Why would you want to be with someone who doesn't accept you or has issues with your surgery?

Most people want the person they love to be healthy.

Years before my surgery, I'd been involved with someone who didn't have an issue with me having Crohn's disease. When I wrote and told him about my surgery and how much better my life was, he never responded. Again, I realized those were his issues, not mine.

There are products available now to help people feel more confident during intimacy, such as wraps and "intimate pouches," that keep your ostomy bag supported and flat against your stomach.

Ostomy surgery gives you back what your disease took away. It gives you a chance to live your life to the fullest. So, go and explore life and all it has to offer. Go and have fun under the covers!

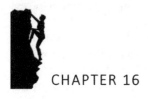

CHAPTER 16

In the End: Insights Gained

Bad things happen; that's a fact. The important thing is how we deal with the situation, and what we ultimately learn about ourselves.

I'm grateful for Crohn's disease and ostomy surgery. I know that might sound strange—after all, why would I be grateful for a disease that caused such trauma in my life? Why am I grateful for a surgery that is still whispered about and viewed as negatively life-altering?

My journey to gratitude didn't happen immediately, but rather, over a long period of time. It started when my father said I would be able to help others because of what I was going through. I had no way of knowing how powerful his answer would become.

Our society is uneasy about discussing bathroom habits. We're taught that it isn't acceptable to discuss diarrhea in "polite company." We use euphemisms to describe what goes on in the privacy of a bathroom, and we laugh nervously when talking about problems "below the belt." Even worse, some people make off-color jokes about a life-saving surgery simply because it deals with our colon. Healing can only begin when feelings can be openly shared.

Crohn's disease and ostomy surgery have taken me down paths I never would have traveled otherwise. They allowed me to discover talents I didn't know I possessed. They helped me meet amazing individuals who made a lasting impression on my life.

I began writing, and found I had a gift for words. Gone was the fear that I wouldn't like myself after ostomy surgery. I began to speak for those who couldn't, and I refused to take no for an answer from Alex, the producer at the *Sally Jessy Raphael Show*. Because of that tenacity, in 1989 there was a frank discussion about Crohn's disease, ulcerative colitis, and ostomy surgery on national television!

I've shared my story with public relations companies, customer service representatives, countless medical and nursing students, and practicing nurses. I worked with my state representative in Washington to pass a restroom access bill so individuals with certain medical conditions couldn't be told that "the bathrooms are for employees only."

I followed my gut feeling that the brown-colored IBD & Ostomy Awareness Ribbon would take off. This campaign to dispel bowel disease's negative image has gained ground, and a brown ribbon with a red jewel in the center has been sent to individuals all over the world. The ribbon's tagline of "it's more than a ribbon, it's a movement" is that and more.

Thirty years after my ostomy surgery, I've made peace with Crohn's disease. Gone are the days when I was in such denial about having a chronic illness that I would rebel by not taking my medication. Gone are the days when I was too embarrassed or afraid to discuss what was happening to my body. Gone are the days when I lived life wondering where the closest bathroom was, afraid to leave my home.

I no longer resent Crohn's disease, and I don't miss my colon or rectum. My stoma reaffirms that I am a gutsy, strong survivor.

I can also appreciate how an ostomy is quite a time-saver, since anyone who has had ostomy surgery excels at multi-tasking. We can give a presentation to a group of individuals and have a bowel movement at the same time!

I've learned that I'm not my disease or my stoma. I've learned to concentrate on what I can accomplish, and on the importance of having friends who accept me as I am. When I discovered what made me laugh, the depression that enveloped me receded enough for me to have hope that I would recover.

In the middle of a crisis, it's difficult to see what benefits this situation might ultimately bring us, and what gifts we might receive if we're willing to see the incident in a different light. When we view a major life event as a way to learn about ourselves, our perception shifts, and we gain a different perspective that can lead to growth and gratitude.

If you have IBD or are facing ostomy surgery, I hope sharing my story gives you the strength and courage to know that you're not alone. You don't have to suffer shame or embarrassment in silence.

Your new normal will be different; I won't deny that. You will feel frightened, and you'll wonder how long it will take before you will feel comfortable changing your pouching system on your own, or looking at your body. You will wonder if intimacy will be possible, and if someone will ever find you attractive.

It will take time to figure out which pouching system works best, and that can only happen by trying different products. Yes, there will be times when the seal on the wafer fails or your peristomal skin gets irritated. You might be afraid to leave the comfort of your home, fearing an accident. You may even wish you weren't alive.

Everyone who has gone through ostomy surgery has experienced these feelings, and the only way to get to the other side is to acknowledge them. Grieve the loss of your colon. Give yourself time. Cry when you need to, and keep the Kleenex box close by.

You *can* live life to the fullest without a colon and rectum, and you'll never have to go through another colonoscopy again. Everybody poops. You'll just do it a little differently!

Additional Perspectives

ADDITIONAL PERSPECTIVES

*What I Know for Sure: Thoughts from
an Ostomy Nurse and Patient*   80

Serving a Unique Community   88

What I Know for Sure: Thoughts from an Ostomy Nurse and Patient

By Joanna Joy Burgess, BSN, RN, CWOCN

Everyone experiences pivotal moments that direct the course of their lives. Some moments send you in a completely different direction than where you were headed only moments before.

For me, that moment came in December of 1965, the month after I turned three. My mother noticed blood in my urine. What was suspected as a simple urinary tract infection turned out to be a rare form of bladder cancer, a type of sarcoma called rhabdomyo-sarcoma.

The surgeons at Boston Children's Hospital grimly and realistically informed my parents that children don't survive this type of cancer, but were willing to give me a 10 percent chance if they proceeded with investigational chemotherapy, cobalt radiation therapy, and bladder removal with the creation of an ileal conduit (urostomy).

I did survive, but due to the radiation therapy, I suffered complications throughout my life, including colitis, which resulted in a colostomy in 1994. Although my body underwent many challenges, my desire and determination to become a nurse never wavered. My career started out in pediatrics at Duke University Medical Center in 1985, and I eventually made my way into the holistic field of nursing, studying massage and healing-touch therapy.

Woven throughout my nursing career was my ongoing story of survival and what my family had to face in taking care of a little girl with an ostomy. I was treated at a time when there were no ostomy nurses at Boston Children's Hospital. My parents relate stories of the nurses being frightened to care for me. On the day of my discharge, my father was handed a brown paper bag with a few ostomy supplies, simple instructions, and a phone number to call to order more. My parents felt alone in my care, and they were. Fumbling through and learning to navigate a seven-piece pouching system was not easy, but we learned through trial and error and I could even manage it on my own by the time I was in the first grade.

In 2005, I reached a place of internal confidence and decided to study the field of wound and ostomy nursing. I soon realized this work would touch me deeply and be an ongoing mirror of what I faced as a child. I am honored to touch the lives of people who have encountered life-altering illnesses that at first seemed unimaginable, and see them learn to adapt and live very well—beyond what they ever thought possible. For many, life is even better and more fulfilling. Such is the case with Lois Fink.

I had the good fortune of meeting Lois when the Wound, Ostomy, and Continence Nurses Society® asked us to speak at their national conference in the summer of 2013. We soon realized the healing power of this connection. I was living in North Carolina, and Lois was living in Seattle. For the next six months we shared our stories, which became the foundation for our talk titled, "What Patients Wish Their Nurses Knew." Through our long-distance conversations, Lois and I realized that although we had traveled a different journey toward ostomy surgery, we both came from the same era of care, which created a bond. We were just two "girls" who felt alone in our experiences, but who finally came together and are now forever connected. Lois has brought a different quality of determination and spunk into my life, along with a lot of humor! I will always be grateful for our friendship.

As an ostomy nurse, I have had the opportunity to see patients in a wide variety of settings, from pre-operative visits, to immediately after ostomy surgery, to clinic visits for follow-up assessments, and at UOAA (United Ostomy Associations of America) support groups and conferences. I also meet with other ostomy nurses regularly, and know the challenges they face when caring for patients. I often see myself as a bridge between the patient and caregiver worlds, and I walk back and forth across that bridge daily, bringing information to both sides with the hope that there will be better understanding of each other's needs.

From my years of ostomy nursing, I would like to share the top three things I know for sure.

1. Ostomy Surgery Strengthens You as a Person

The emotional impact of facing ostomy surgery and then learning to live with an ostomy can unleash the gamut of emotions. Just recently at a patient-support group for those who had survived bladder cancer, I heard a psychiatrist say, "A traumatic incident has more to do with the future than it has to do with the past."

For me that was certainly true—anyone facing ostomy surgery, whether they're young or old, always wants to know, What does this mean for my life as I look forward? Will I be able to function as I once did? Will I be able to work? Will I be able to have an intimate relationship? Will people be accepting of me? Will I even be able to *be* me?

It is the transformation of the once-known into the new unknown that is the ostomy patient's new future. The fear of the unknown can only be eradicated by learning from those who've undergone the same experience.

I encourage my patients, and the family members who care for them, to write down their questions and fears related to ostomy surgery. We then discuss them one by one. The more information a patient has, the more comfortable they become. For some patients, I recommend counseling. A licensed clinical social worker has the skills to help a patient create the life tools for navigating the unknown, especially for those with fears of introducing their ostomy into a new or existing relationship.

It's important for patients to seek the resources they need to understand and move through the grieving process related to ostomy surgery. Grief is a natural process related to loss, and we ebb and flow through the stages as we emotionally heal. It's helpful to have someone affirm feelings of loss and show the path to acceptance and adaptation. I've had many patients who were initially devastated at the thought of ostomy surgery, but who eventually went on to become mentors to others facing the same surgery.

Growing up, it was always important for me to have heroes in my life. In an age where the world was not as connected as it is now, my family didn't know anyone who'd had ostomy surgery, so my heroes were people who faced other physical challenges. I looked up to Joni Eareckson Tada, the singer and artist who became a quadriplegic after a diving accident but went on to have a career and marriage. As a little girl, I found hope for those same things in my own life. Today, I have many heroes who have been through ostomy surgery. I have met, to list a few, teachers, military personal, athletes, and models who are living well and thriving with an ostomy. I encourage all new and established ostomates to join support groups (UOAA affiliates or online groups) so they know they're not alone on this journey. Once ostomates learn to care for their ostomy, move through their grief, and realize they can in fact handle it, they realize their strength in every aspect of life. Having an ostomy gave me the determination to become a nurse in order to help others, the assertiveness to be a patient advocate, and the skills to adapt and meet other life challenges along the way. Ostomy surgery gave me so much more than it ever took away.

2. Messes and Skin Issues Are Part of the Package

My husband and I had known each other only a few months when we decided I should meet his family. This entailed a trip from North Carolina to Tennessee. We stopped at a restaurant and each ordered a Reuben sandwich, which caused one of the biggest ostomy messes I have ever had, commonly referred to in the ostomy population as a "blowout." My husband handled the situation beautifully and kindly gave me his shirt, and off I went to a roadside bathroom to clean up.

I always tell patients to be prepared for messes and learn from your mistakes. I no longer eat a Reuben on the road, and I always have plenty of paper towels, extra supplies, and a change of clothes just in case. In the moment, a mess can seem like the end of the world and can certainly trigger anger and tears, as they always seem to come at the worst time. They often make for comical stories later on, and life does go on.

Studies and research have shown that most ostomy patients will at some point have issues related to the skin breaking down. Skin problems can result from a multitude of scenarios. The most common include a poorly fitting or improper pouching system (which can cause ongoing leakage of urine or stool), allergic reactions to products, or the misuse of ostomy products.

To avoid damage to the skin, it is important for patients to seek advice from an ostomy nurse as soon as a problem manifests. One of my first ostomy-clinic patients was a man who had been using the same pouching system for 50 years. He came to me stating that for a year, he'd had problems with the pouch not working, and his skin had begun to break down. I determined that with age, his body contours were no longer the same, and he required a different type of pouch. Change was hard, but I worked with him until he found success with an appropriate system for his changing body type. To find the best pouching system, an ostomy nurse will assess the stoma and the skin around it while you exhibit different positions (standing, sitting, lying down, and bending).

For patients who do not have access to an ostomy nurse in the hospital or in an outpatient setting, I recommend going to the support network of their supply manufacturer. Most companies that manufacture ostomy supplies have a team of professionals who can troubleshoot problems. It isn't the same as having an in-person assessment, so it's vital to be as descriptive as possible. It's also important to describe your stoma (round, oval, budded, flush to the skin) and the skin around your stoma (smooth, creases, mounds, lumps) to the person trying to help you. I encourage you to know your stoma in the same way an ostomy nurse would, for it will serve you well in seeking assistance and will help avoid those messes and skin problems!

3. Ostomy Surgery Is Life-Altering, Life-Changing, and Life-Giving

I've met a few new ostomates whose first words to me were along the lines of, "Death would be an improvement over what I am living with." Some are ready to "hibernate" and become reclusive. Then I tell them my story, and soon I see the signs of hope returning to their eyes. This is the real gift of being an ostomy nurse who has an ostomy.

Having ostomy surgery gave me my life back twice. The first was the choice my parents made to save my life. The second was my choice to be free of ongoing pain and incontinence from radiation-induced colitis. If I had the choice to give anything back in life, it would not be my ostomies or the cancer that lead to them. I might give back the poor choices in relationships I made prior to meeting my husband, the nursing instructor in college who told me if I wasn't good at math I should reconsider nursing as my major, the endless whispers growing up of children wanting to know what was wrong with me because I walked with a limp, or my inability to have children. But I don't think I would give those back either.

I believe everything in life shapes us, and a change of perception is often our miracle. Poor choices led me to the right choice and I met my husband; doubts from teachers made me all the more determined to succeed; whispers from children caused me to seek out friends I could trust and depend on; and I've learned to seek out and love the child who remains in everyone–especially with my fearful ostomy patients, whom I take under my wing like a mother. To date, I've had my ostomy for fifty-one years, and I am forever grateful. I believe the hundreds of ostomy patients I've counseled over the years would agree!

—Joanna Joy Burgess, BSN, RN, CWOCN

Serving a Unique Community

By Ed Pfueller, Communications and Outreach Manager, UOAA

People with an ostomy are unique, but they are not alone. Ostomy surgery is performed for a wide variety of reasons. It can sustain a newborn in the first days of life, or it can be the last resort to treat a disease that could otherwise end a person's life. It can be planned for and elective, or completely unexpected. It can be temporary, or for life. It can be the result of war injuries in a foreign land or a trauma at home. Organs such as the bladder, colon, small intestine, kidneys, or liver can require ostomy surgery. Even stoma size and placement varies from person to person.

Yet there is a common bond among people living with an ostomy that is undeniable, and there is one national organization working for a better quality of life for them all.

The United Ostomy Associations of America Inc. (UOAA) was founded in 2005 to work toward a society where people with ostomies and intestinal or urinary diversions are universally accepted and supported socially, economically, medically, and psychologically.

The organization was created to fill a void left by the dissolution of United Ostomy Association (UOA), and seeks to maintain a legacy of over forty-three years of support for the ostomy community. The UOAA continues to use UOA's symbol of the phoenix, which represents "rising from the ashes of disease."

The UOAA is an association of more than 300 affiliated support groups (ASGs) organized by volunteers throughout the United States. It provides the opportunity for local, in-person support. People living with ostomies or continent diversions are welcome before or after surgery, along with their caregivers, friends, and family.

The UOAA exists to serve people living with an ostomy, wherever they may be. They make quality ostomy information and resources available online and accept calls from all those with questions about ostomies and continent diversions, and make every effort to connect callers to the resources they need.

When the ostomy community needs a voice on Capitol Hill or in their statehouse, the UOAA is there to fight for the medical needs and rights of this diverse community. Stigmas surrounding ostomy surgery may still emerge, but the UOAA is there to provide a true reflection of an active community. It is an organization dedicated to those it serves.

Trusted Resources and Support

Quality peer support has the power to change lives. Connecting with others who embrace an active life with an ostomy or continent diversion can be the spark many people need to begin thriving in life after surgery. Affiliated support groups around the country provide a safe space for ostomates to learn, ask questions, or simply enjoy the camaraderie of a welcoming ostomy community.

Some people find confidence in their "new normal" lives and choose to stay in their support groups to pay it forward. Hard-working volunteers spend countless hours making sure this service is available in their local communities. UOAA President Susan

Burns, of St. Louis, is just one example of a support-group leader who sought to serve even more people through national leadership in UOAA.

"Support meetings were vital as I began a new chapter in my life and recovery," Burns remembers. "I knew I wanted to help the next people in need."

On a national level, the organization is run by a volunteer board of directors spread out across the United States and supported by a small staff.

Recognizing that not everyone lives near or is able to attend a support group, the UOAA serves those living with an ostomy and continent diversion wherever they may be. In this Internet age, a plethora of medical information is a keystroke away. To cut through the noise, the UOAA provides independent and medically-reviewed educational information.

Surgery-specific, new-patient guides for colostomy, ileostomy, urostomy, and continent diversion are available online and mailed by request to both health-care professionals and individuals who have had or may have ostomy surgery. Adjusting to life with an ostomy can be a challenge for many. The UOAA helps to ease this transition with online guides on diet and nutrition, sexuality and intimacy, skin care, and other information critical for maintaining a good quality of life.

The community can also seek answers to questions by posting on UOAA's online discussion board. A wide variety of topics are discussed and archived in this forum. An active and supportive Facebook community with curated ostomy content is also available for all. Moreover, UOAA's monthly e-newsletter serves to inform the ostomy community about the latest news, events, and national advocacy efforts. The UOAA website is www.ostomy.org.

The Phoenix Magazine is the official publication

of the UOAA and the premiere magazine for ostomy information. It is filled with lifelong learning and inspiring stories from the ostomy community, and is available by subscription both online and by mail.

UOAA conferences also provide an opportunity for the national ostomy community to gather for education, camaraderie, and support. Renowned experts and leaders in the ostomy community seek to impart their knowledge to all who attend.

Information is power, and with it, people can then be their own self-advocates in navigating personal health-care needs.

Speaking Up for the Community

At a national level, perhaps no function of the UOAA affects more people than that of its advocacy program. The UOAA represents the voice of the ostomy community on the issues that matter in maintaining the highest quality of life for all those living with an ostomy. For example, when access to ostomy supplies is threatened by proposals such as those related to Medicare competitive bidding, the UOAA is there.

The UOAA works to educate legislators on why ostomy products are not a one-size-fits-all product. As the advocacy program grows, it's connecting directly with individuals who have powerful stories to tell about the consequences of restrictions on prescribed ostomy products. Together, personal stories can have a profound impact. We join with allies whenever possible to ensure that the most effective methods are undertaken in communications with lawmakers.

Issues important to the ostomy community can pop up from year to year or be ongoing. Restrictions to ostomy supplies on a national level, such as with Medicare, can in turn influence private insurers and state marketplace health plans. Only three states currently have mandates for health-care plans to cover ostomy supplies. There's always more work to be done.

The UOAA also works with the Transportation Safety Administration (TSA) to ease the air-travel experience for ostomates everywhere. As a result, complaints with the screening process are rare, and when they happen, they're taken very seriously. Online, www.ostomy.org provides travel tips, TSA information, and a traveler's card for all to utilize. The travel card can be printed and handed to security personnel at the beginning of the screening process to discreetly inform them that you have an ostomy, and can also be used on the plane for communicating the possible medical need for bathroom access during a restricted time in flight.

Education and awareness remain an important part of national-advocacy success. Despite progress in recent years, stigma and misinformation about ostomy surgery are still prevalent. Individuals have contacted the UOAA office with stories of being denied access to the swimming facility of their choice, for instance. By producing an online toolkit that can be used to educate both swimmers and pool person-nel, the UOAA is working to put an end to these incidents.

Ostomy Awareness Day brings together the di-verse ostomy community on the first Saturday of October. The annual event was initiated by the organization in 2010. The day is a chance for ostomates to be proud, celebrate accomplishments, and educate people everywhere about the needs of the ostomy community.

Outreach for the Future

Erasing any stigmas about ostomy surgery is at the heart of the UOAA's vision for the future of the ostomy community. It's a busy world, and people need to be reached wherever they spend time. Increasingly, that is on social media. These outlets allow the organization to reach people perhaps hearing about United Ostomy Associations of America for the first time. Engaging younger populations early on in their ostomy journey will hopefully strengthen the future of the organization.

The future looks bright. Many of the younger generations are embracing their ostomies and speaking very openly about their lives in public forums, both online and in person. They are reaching a society that has traditionally held a narrow worldview of who has a "colostomy bag." The UOAA supports this new generation as it works to erode stigmas.

Part of the UOAA's outreach includes fun awareness events that bring the community together. The Run for Resilience Ostomy 5k events provide positive exposure for the ostomy community and the active lifestyle that many living with an ostomy lead. An idea started by two Certified Wound, Ostomy, and Continence nurses in Durham, North Carolina has now spread to locations across the United States, and also to London, England. Local volunteers organize the events and are passionate about the cause. They are supported by the UOAA's staff and board members.

The power of the Run for Resilience events is magnified when they harness the energy of ostomy supporters on social networks. All new initiatives hope to grow the community of support that the

UOAA has built since its inception in 2005. Social media, when responsibly managed, can have a positive influence in building communities of support in new ways.

An Organization for Everyone

The supporters and volunteers of the UOAA are the backbone of its success. They are the reason the organization has been able to help countless people live full and productive lives with an ostomy. The United Ostomy Associations of America continues to serve the many people dedicated to its mission of support by being open to all who may benefit from their resources.

—Ed Pfueller, Communications & Outreach
Manager, UOAA

Further Learning

FURTHER LEARNING

Glossary   97

List of Resources   102

Glossary

Common Terms

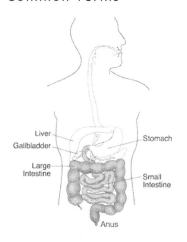

Gastrointestinal (GI) tract: The muscular tube that takes food from the mouth, through the esophagus to the stomach and then the intestines, and expels it via the anus. Its main function is to break food down into nutrients. Food is chewed and moistened in the mouth first. Then, the food is digested by the stomach and small intestine, where fats and carbohydrates are broken down. The small intestine absorbs these nutrients, and the large intestine reabsorbs water back into the body. The remaining waste is expelled via the anus.

Ostomy: A surgically-created opening in the body that is connected to the gastrointestinal or urinary tract. It is used for the discharge of body waste (urine or stool). The opening can be created from the small or large intestine.

Stoma: A word that simply means "opening." A stoma is red and moist, and protrudes like a bud outside the abdomen.

Common Types of Ostomies

The most common types of ostomies are colostomies, ileostomies, and urostomies. These ostomies have no sphincter control, and a bag or pouching system must be worn to collect waste.

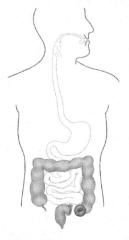

Colostomy: A surgically-created opening on the abdomen in which a piece of the colon (large intestine) is brought outside the abdominal wall to create a stoma. A colostomy is needed when a portion of the colon or rectum is removed due to a disease process or damaged area of the colon. A colostomy may be temporary or permanent, depending on the medical reason for the surgery. The stoma is usually located on the left side of the abdomen.

Ileostomy: A surgically-created opening on the abdomen in which a piece of the small intestine (usually the end of the ileum) is brought outside the abdominal wall to create a stoma. Ileostomies may be temporary or permanent, and are a result of the removal of a section of the small intestine or all or part of the colon. This stoma is located on the right side of the abdomen.

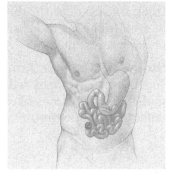

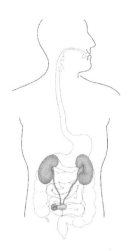

Urostomy (ileal conduit): A surgical procedure that diverts urine away from a diseased or defective bladder, or drains urine from the kidneys if the bladder has been removed (most commonly due to cancer). The ureters are attached to an isolated section of the small intestine (the ileum), creating a passageway (conduit) that is brought outside the abdomen to create a stoma. Urine will no longer be eliminated from the urethra, but will drain out the stoma into a pouch or bag. This stoma is located on the right side of the abdomen.

Other Types of Ostomies

Nephrostomy: A surgical procedure in which a nephrostomy tube is inserted through the skin and into the kidney to allow urine to drain into a pouch or bag. It is usually necessary when there is a blockage impeding urine flow.

Cecostomy: A surgical procedure to create a small opening in the abdomen to the cecum (the beginning of the large intestine). It allows a tube (catheter) to be placed for irrigating the colon. It is used as an alternative to an enema to empty the colon.

Gastrostomy: An opening created through the skin and into the stomach. A tube may be placed for venting or drainage, or for a feeding tube that delivers nutritional support directly into the stomach.

Continent diversion procedures: Continence is the ability to control the elimination of urine or stool. Continent diversions are created for voluntary control over urinary and fecal discharge. These diversions do not require a pouching system.

Continent ileostomy (Kock pouch): An ileostomy that drains into a surgically-created pouch or reservoir located in the abdomen and made from loops of the small intestine (ileum). Involuntary discharge of intestinal contents to the outside of the body is prevented by a nipple valve created from the ileum. This method eliminates the need for the patient to wear an external pouch over the stoma. The stoma is catheterized throughout the day to empty the reservoir. A small dressing or bandage is worn over the stoma.

Ileoanal reservoir (J-pouch): A procedure in which the colon and most of the rectum are surgically removed and an internal pouch is formed out of the terminal portion of the small intestine (ileum). An opening at the bottom of this pouch is attached to the anus in a way that the existing anal sphincter muscles can be used for continence. This procedure most often is performed on patients with ulcerative colitis or familial polyposis who have not previously lost their anal sphincters. In addition to the "J" pouch, there are "S" and "W" pouches, depending on the shape of the pouch needed. This is also called an ileoanal anastomosis, endorectal pull-through, pelvic pouch, or ileal pouch anal anastomosis (IPAA).

Continent urinary diversion (Indiana pouch): The creation of an intestinal reservoir with a catheterizable channel that is brought from the reservoir to the skin with creation of a stoma. The channel can be catheterized several times a day to empty the reservoir. The Indiana pouch has become the predominant urinary diversion for patients who desire continence. The intestinal reservoir can be made from a variety of bowel segments.

Orthotopic urinary diversion (neobladder): A surgically-created reservoir (neobladder) that is then anastomosed (connected) to the urethra. This is for those who do not want a stoma and wish to void per the urethra. Reservoirs are typically created from 50 to 60 cm of the ileum.

For more information, visit the United Ostomy Associations of America online at www.ostomy.org.

List of Resources

Crohn's & Colitis Foundation of America, Inc. (CCFA)
733 Third Avenue; Suite 510
New York, NY 10017
800-932-2423
www.ccfa.org
Email: info@ccfa.org

International Ostomy Association (IOA)
800-826-0826
www.ostomyinternational.org
Email: oa@ostomy.org

Ostomy Canada Society
5800 Ambler Drive #210
Mississauga, ON L4W 4J4, Canada
905-212-7111
888-969-9698 (Canada) T–Th 8:30 A.M.–4:30 P.M. EST
www.ostomycanada.ca
Email: info@ostomycanada.ca

United Ostomy Associations of America, Inc. (UOAA)
P.O. Box 525
Kennebunk, ME 04043-0525
800-826-0826
www.ostomy.org
Email: oa@ostomy.org

WOUND, OSTOMY, AND CONTINENCE NURSING CERTIFICATION

Wound, Ostomy, and Continence Nursing Certification Board
555 East Wells Street, Suite 1100
Milwaukee, WI 53202-3823
888-496-2622
www.wocncb.org
Email: info@wocncb.org

WOUND, OSTOMY, AND CONTINENCE NURSES SOCIETY

Wound, Ostomy, and Continence Nurses Society®
1120 Rt. 73, Suite 200
Mount Laurel, NJ 08054
888-224-9626
www.wocn.org
Email: wocn_info@wocn.org

MEDICAL/OSTOMY SUPPLY COMPANIES

(This is a partial listing)

Byram Healthcare
120 Bloomingdale Road, Suite 301
White Plains, NY 10605
877-902-9726
www.byramhealthcare.com
They offer a discount for cash purchases.

Edgepark Medical Supplies (a division of Cardinal Health)
1810 Summit Commerce Park
Twinsburg, OH 44087
888-394-5375
www.edgepark.com

Nu-Hope Laboratories, Inc.
12640 Branford Street
Pacoima, CA 91331
800-899-5017
www.nu-hope.com

Osto Group
3500 45th Street, Suite 16A
West Palm Beach, FL 32407
877-678-6690
www.ostogroup.org
Free ostomy supplies for those in the United States without Medicare or other health insurance. There is a small charge for handling cost and postage.

Shield HealthCare
27911 Franklin Parkway
Valencia, CA 91355
800-765-8775
www.shieldhealthcare.com

Stomabags
7420 West 18 Lane
Miami, FL 33014
855-828-1444
www.stomabags.com
Discount ostomy supplies for the under- or non-insured.

Total HomeCare Supplies
27911 Franklin Parkway
Valencia, CA 91355
866-376-4950
www.totalhomecaresupplies.com
Supplies offered at a discount.

OSTOMY MANUFACTURERS/COMPANIES

(This is a partial listing)

Coloplast Corporation
1601 West River Road North
Minneapolis, MN 55411
800-788-0293
www.coloplast.com

ConvaTec, Inc.
211 American Avenue
Greensboro, NC 27409
800-422-8811 (M–F 8:30 A.M.-7:00 P.M.)
www.convatec.com
Email: cic@convatec.com

Hollister Incorporated
2000 Hollister Drive
Libertyville, IL 60048-3781
800-323-4060
www.hollister.com
Products: 888-740-8899
Secure Start™ Services: 888-808-7456
Illustrations courtesy of Hollister Incorporated, Libertyville, Illinois.
Hollister Incorporated is not responsible for the content of this material.

MEDIA AND PUBLICATIONS

OstomyConnection
www.ostomyconnection.com

The Phoenix Ostomy Magazine
800-750-9311
www.phoenixuoaa.org

ONLINE DISCUSSION/SUPPORT GROUPS

ColonTown
www.colontown.org

Inspire Community
www.inspire.com/groups/ostomy
Users can join the site, create a profile, and participate in community discussions online. There are many other condition-specific communities on the site as well.

United Ostomy Associations of America, Inc.
www.uoaa.org/forum/index.php

VeganOstomy
www.veganostomy.ca

NUTRITION

USDA Center for Nutrition Policy and Promotion
3101 Park Center Drive, Room 1034
Alexandria, VA 22302-1594
703-305-7600
www.choosemyplate.gov

Food and Nutrition Information Center
National Agricultural Library, ARS, USDA
301-504-5414, M-F 8:30 A.M.-4:30 P.M. EST
Email: www.fnic@usda.gov

SEXUALITY

United Ostomy Associations of America, Inc. (UOAA)
www.ostomy.org
"Intimacy, Sexuality and an Ostomy" booklet is available only online as a guidebook under "Ostomy Info" section.

Gay and Lesbian Ostomates
773-286-4005
www.glo-uoaa.org

TRAVEL

Centers for Disease Control and Prevention (CDC)
1600 Clifton Road
Atlanta, GA 30329-4027
800-232-4636
www.cdc.gov/travel

International Association for Medical Assistance to
Travelers (IAMAT)
716-754-4883
www.iamat.org
Email: info@iamat.org

Transportation Security Agency (TSA)
U.S. Department of Homeland Security
866-289-9673
www.tsa.gov
Contact: tsa.gov/contact/contact-forms
*Current information about travel security rules and
regulations for travelers with disabilities and medical
conditions.*

U.S. Department of State
www.travel.state.gov
Information on travel alerts for specific countries.

*Yes We Can! Advice on Traveling with an Ostomy and
Tips for Everyday Living* by Barbara Kupfer
Chandler House Press, 2000

EXERCISE

National Institute on Aging (NIA)
800-222-2225
www.nia.nih.gov/health/publication/exercise-physical-activity/introduction

Run for Resilience Ostomy 5K Events
www.ostomy5k.org

INTIMATE WEAR

Awestomy
800-269-2830
www.awestomy.com
Email: info@awestomy.com
This company donates 15 percent of sales to a nonprofit company each month through their Give A Sh*t program.

My Heart Ties
3910 Caughey Road, Suite 140
Erie, PA 16506
888-338-TIES
www.myheartties.com

Ostomysecrets
877-613-6246
www.ostomysecrets.com
Email: info@ostomysecrets.com

Vanilla Blush
Unit 43 Dalmarnock Road
Bridgeton, Glasgow, G40 4LA
www.vblush.com

SUPPORT BELTS/POUCH COVERS

C&S Ostomy Pouch Covers
2214 Cloras Street
North Port, FL 34287
877-754-9913
www.cspouchcovers.com

PouchWear
2554 W. 16th Street, Suite 136
Yuma, AZ 85364-4229
844-768-2493
www.ostomybagholder.com
Email: support@ostomybagholder.com

Stealthbelt, Inc.
210 West Oakland Avenue, Suite D
Johnson City, TN 37604
800-237-4491
www.stealthbelt.com

INSURANCE AND WORK ISSUES

Equal Opportunity Commission
800-669-4000
www.eeoc.gov
Information on work-discrimination issues.

US. Department of Labor
200 Constitution Avenue NW
Washington, DC 20210
866-487-2365
www.dol.gov
Search for HIPAA (Health Insurance Portability and Accountability Act).

CHILDREN

Shadow Buddies Foundation
14700 West 107th Street, Suite 100
Lenexa, KS 66215
913-642-4646
www.shadowbuddies.org
Email: buddies@shadowbuddies.org
Dolls with ostomies.

TEENS

Youth Rally
www.youthrally.org
A community that allows adolescents living with bowel and bladder conditions to meet each other in an atmosphere that promotes self-confidence and independence.

About the Author

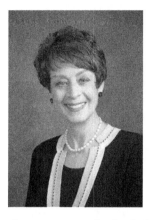

"If sharing my story helps someone, then what I went through had meaning and purpose."

Lois Fink was dismissed and ignored by the medical community for nearly two years as she battled an undiagnosed disease as a teenager. An emergency appendectomy when she was a senior in high school solved the mystery: she had Crohn's disease. She weighed just 62 pounds by the time the disease was discovered.

Ostomy surgery at age thirty-six gave her back everything Crohn's disease had taken away: a full, active life free from pain, embarrassment, and shame.

Today, Lois is an internationally-renowned inspirational speaker, patient advocate, and writer. She lives in Fort Collins, Colorado, where she enjoys the sunshine, the Rocky Mountains, and the friends she's made since leaving Seattle.

Photo by Gail Ann Photography.

Speaking Engagements

Lois Fink is an internationally-renowned inspirational speaker who discusses subject matter we normally don't want to hear about—intense abdominal pain, diarrhea, bowel incontinence, her fear of having an accident in public, and the need to know where the nearest bathroom is at all times—with honesty and laser precision. She takes you along for the ride as she talks about her lifelong battle with Crohn's disease and what she's learned along the way.

RAVE REVIEWS

"Marvelous, moving, funny, passionate, a gifted speaker, beautiful . . . what a phenomenal woman."

—First-year medical student, U. of Colorado's Anschutz Medical Campus

"Lois Fink was the best speaker of the day. I plan to use her recommendations when working with this very special group of patients and their families."

—Participant, U. of Washington's Update in Medical-Surgical Nursing Conference

CONTACT

To hire Lois for a speaking engagement, visit www.couragetakesguts.com or email fink.lois@gmail.com.

Made in the USA
Monee, IL
30 August 2021

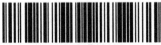